"How I wish I'd had this book when I suffered from postpartum obses[sions]. Pregnant and postpartum moms need to know that perinatal anxiety [is] treatable, and that there's no need to continue suffering. It is infinitely comforting to read such a calm and objective discussion of the symptoms of this illness and to be given practical self-help tools to move toward recovery."

—Katherine Stone, editor of *Postpartum Progress*, the most widely-read blog on perinatal mood and anxiety disorders, and board member of Postpartum Support International

"Finally, a workbook for *anxiety* during pregnancy and the postpartum period! Wiegartz and Gyoerkoe have adapted the powerful and scientifically proven techniques of cognitive behavioral therapy into tools that new moms and mothers-to-be can use to overcome the most common anxiety-related problems and reclaim this special time of life. Readers will learn about anxiety from the clear explanations and develop skills using the innovative worksheets in this book. Every expecting parent (moms and dads) can benefit from this workbook."

—Jonathan S. Abramowitz, Ph.D., ABPP, professor and director of the Anxiety and Stress Disorders Clinic at the University of North Carolina at Chapel Hill

"This superb book, written by two experienced clinical psychologists, offers practical, scientifically proven methods for helping expectant and new mothers overcome anxiety problems, such as excessive worry, obsessions, and panic attacks. I highly recommend this book to all expectant or new mothers and fathers—who are seeking relief from anxiety."

—Steven Taylor, Ph.D., ABPP, psychiatry professor at the University of British Columbia and author of *Treating Health Anxiety* and *The Clinician's Guide to PTSD*

"This book is destined to become the new bible for any expectant or new mom suffering from serious anxiety. It brings state-of-the-art breakthroughs in anxiety treatment to women in a clear, compassionate, practical, and user-friendly self-help format."

—Valerie Davis Raskin, MD, author of *This Isn't What I Expected*

"New mothers, fathers, and their families will appreciate this easy-to-read and instructive book on how to manage anxiety before and after the birth of a child. *The Pregnancy and Postpartum Anxiety Workbook* explains the likely sources and expressions of anxiety during this phase of life and provides specific strategies for reducing anxious thoughts and behaviors. The chapter on fathers in the final section will appeal to dads who are also struggling with strong emotions as a new baby enters the picture."

—Gail Steketee, Ph.D., dean and professor at Boston University's School of Social Work and author of *Overcoming Obsessive-Compulsive Disorder*

"This book provides pregnant women with the support and hope they need during one of the most amazing experiences in life—pregnancy. The book includes a matter-of-fact discussion of specific techniques which help with anxiety during the pregnancy and postpartum period."

—Jerald S. Goldstein, MD, reproductive endocrinologist and infertility specialist at Fertility Specialists of Dallas

The Pregnancy & Postpartum Anxiety Workbook

Practical Skills to Help You Overcome Anxiety, Worry, Panic Attacks, Obsessions, and Compulsions

PAMELA S. WIEGARTZ, PH.D.
KEVIN L. GYOERKOE, PSY.D.

New Harbinger Publications, Inc.

For Jackson, my greatest joy and daily wonder
—PSW

For Mom
—KLG

Distributed in Canada by Raincoast Books

Copyright © 2009 by Pamela S. Wiegartz and Kevin L. Gyoerkoe
New Harbinger Publications, Inc.
5674 Shattuck Avenue
Oakland, CA 94609
www.newharbinger.com

Cover design by Amy Shoup; Text design by Amy Shoup and Michele Waters-Kermes;
Acquired by Tesilya Hanauer; Edited by Karen O'Donnell Stein

All Rights Reserved. Printed in the United States of America.

FSC
Mixed Sources
Product group from well-managed
forests and other controlled sources

Cert no. SW-COC-002283
www.fsc.org
© 1996 Forest Stewardship Council

11   10   09

10   9   8   7   6   5   4   3   2   1   First printing

Contents

PART 3
Applying Cognitive Behavioral Therapy to Specific Anxiety Problems

PART 4
Maintaining Positive Changes

Acknowledgments

We'd like to thank Jess Beebe, Tesilya Hanauer, and Karen O'Donnell Stein, our editors at New Harbinger Publications. You are all a true pleasure to work with. We are grateful for your support, enthusiasm, and insightful contributions to this book.

We'd also like to thank Dr. Laura Miller for her expert comments on early drafts of this project. Thank you, Laura—we appreciate your time, your valuable feedback, and your tireless advocacy for women's mental health.

Of course, we also want to thank our patients—new moms and moms to be suffering from anxiety—for allowing us into your world and giving us the opportunity to work with you. Your courage and persistence in conquering anxiety are an inspiration.

And finally, we thank our families for their encouragement and patience during the many late nights we spent writing. Without you, this book would not have been possible.

Foreword

Just about every mother-to-be has at least *some* worries about being pregnant, giving birth, and parenting. Most of us worry about whether our babies will be healthy, whether we can manage the pain of labor, or whether we will be the type of mother we want to be. These are normal anxieties, and most of the time, they don't paralyze us or cause us to panic. But in some cases, anxiety and anxious thoughts during pregnancy can become frequent, severe, and highly distressing. If left unchecked, severe anxiety can interfere with the joy of bringing a new life into the world and can make pregnancy and birth more difficult physically as well as emotionally.

Fortunately, there are effective strategies to reduce severe anxiety during and after pregnancy. As a reproductive psychiatrist, I've worked with hundreds of pregnant and postpartum women at the University of Illinois at Chicago Women's Clinic, and I have seen the tremendous benefits reaped by women who learn these strategies and conquer their anxiety symptoms. Over the years, many women have asked if there was a book they could read to help them learn techniques that work for pregnancy and postpartum anxiety. Now I can finally say yes! Pamela Wiegartz and Kevin Gyoerkoe wrote *The Pregnancy and Postpartum Anxiety Workbook* for women who are planning a pregnancy, already pregnant, or postpartum and want to tame their anxieties or prevent severe anxiety from happening in the first place.

As you read *The Pregnancy and Postpartum Anxiety Workbook*, you will learn how to assess your own anxiety symptoms. You will practice relaxation techniques that are safe and manageable while you're pregnant or sore from having given birth. You will become skilled at identifying anxious thoughts and knowing how to defuse them. You will improve your ability to solve problems and prioritize your time. If you have symptoms such as panic attacks, obsessive thoughts, worries, and post-traumatic stress reactions, you will learn strategies specifically geared to these symptoms. For all of these skills, you will find clear explanations, specific instructions, and checklists to help you keep track. There are lots of suggestions for your partner, too, so your partner can understand your anxiety and help you in effective ways.

In addition to being experts on anxiety disorders and their treatment, Drs. Wiegartz and Gyoerkoe are parents themselves. They get it! They know learning anxiety management skills can be difficult under any circumstances, but especially while you're pregnant or during the busy, exhausting weeks and months of new motherhood. The techniques they recommend take practice, but they are realistic and they work. As you read this workbook, you will feel the authors' confident, encouraging empathy come through. You will find yourself becoming more and more skilled at managing your anxiety, and you will no longer feel alone.

Laura J. Miller, MD
Director, Women's Mental Health Program
University of Illinois at Chicago

Introduction

Congratulations! If you've picked up this book, you are, or will soon be, a new mother. Welcome to one of the most wonderful experiences imaginable. Having a child is truly the pinnacle of happiness. However, it can also be fraught with anxiety, fear, and worry. What if something goes wrong? What if I'm not a good mom? How will I handle it? If you've picked up this workbook, you are already familiar with the litany of worries that can accompany motherhood and cast a shadow over this amazing time in your life.

Or maybe someone you care about—your spouse, a family member, or a friend—is struggling with anxiety. Perhaps you're a treatment provider hoping to learn new ways to help your patients. Whatever the case, we're glad you have chosen this book. As clinicians and as parents ourselves, we are deeply committed to the cause of battling anxiety in pregnancy and the postpartum period. Our goal is to bring public awareness, education, and treatment of this all-too-common problem to everyone.

Sadly, recent studies have found that only about one-third of women with anxiety disorders have actually been diagnosed and received treatment (Sampson 2001) and that only about 20 percent of obstetricians (OBs) regularly screen for anxiety during pregnancy (Coleman et al. 2008).

Because you are reading this book, you are already ahead of the game—too many women suffer in silence or don't have access to appropriate treatment. We couldn't count the number of horror stories we've heard from our clients who've been to multiple providers and have undergone many ineffective treatments before finding us. Misdiagnosis, outdated information, inappropriate treatment—the list of problems goes on and on. That's why we wrote *The Pregnancy & Postpartum Anxiety Workbook: Practical Skills to Help You Overcome Anxiety, Worry, Panic Attacks, Obsessions, and Compulsions.*

Featuring research-proven cognitive behavioral therapy (CBT) techniques, this book is the answer for anxious new moms and moms-to-be. We've carefully chosen strategies that work to defeat anxiety—the same strategies we use with our patients—and adapted them to fit the needs of pregnant and postpartum women. Research shows that CBT can effectively lower anxiety during pregnancy and the postpartum period and result in long-lasting gains (Austin et al. 2008). So read on and learn how this book can help *you* overcome your anxiety and calmly and fully experience all that motherhood has to offer!

How to Use This Book

As you read this book, you'll notice that it's made up of four parts. The first part offers background information on anxiety during pregnancy and the postpartum period and explains available treatments. Part 2 will teach you, step-by-step, a variety of research-proven cognitive behavioral techniques that work for anxiety. In this section you'll find the skills and strategies you'll need in order to battle your anxiety. Part 3 addresses specific anxiety problems you may experience, like panic attacks, obsessions and compulsions, worry, and post-traumatic stress. In that section, you will learn how to fine-tune your skills, apply them to these problem areas, and conquer your anxiety once and for all. Part 4 will help you to maintain these positive changes throughout your life.

To help you get the most out of this book, we have a few suggestions:

- Be sure to practice all of the techniques in part 2. Not everyone will respond the same way to each strategy. Try them all until you find the ones that work for you.

- Do the exercises in each chapter. Just like you can't simply pick up a book on dieting and automatically lose weight, you won't beat your anxiety just by reading about it. Pick up your pen or pencil—just like our clients do—and get started!

- Get help if you need it. If you find the strategies too difficult to do on your own, you can use this book in conjunction with therapy to speed your recovery from anxiety. A resource list can be found near the end of this book to help you locate an appropriate therapist who is experienced in treating anxiety.

- Keep at it. Though CBT is fast and effective, anxiety can be a tough foe. It takes time and work to truly master these skills and overcome your anxiety, but the results will be worth it!

From the Authors

Pamela S. Wiegartz, Ph.D.

As a psychologist specializing in the treatment of anxiety for over a decade, I have long held an interest in the worries and fears that accompany pregnancy and the postpartum period—simply because so many of my clients seem to struggle with them. The lack of resources for women to address this very treatable problem still amazes me, and my patients have often said, "You should write a book on this!" When I became a mom, I knew that they were right. I now know firsthand how amazing pregnancy and motherhood can be—and also how scary. That is why we wrote this book—to give pregnant and new moms real strategies to address the anxieties that inevitably go along with a new baby. This book combines years of clinical practice, the latest research findings, and firsthand experience to give you the information and skills you need to enter motherhood on solid ground. Good luck to you on this magnificent journey!

Kevin L. Gyoerkoe, Psy.D.

I'm truly thrilled to bring you this workbook. In my practice, I see every kind of patient suffering from every kind of anxiety problem imaginable. However, one group of patients always stands out—new moms and moms-to-be. Even though anxiety always inflicts unwanted suffering, it seems especially cruel that an anxiety problem would strike during one of the best times of your life. The last thing you want is for anxiety to spoil this special time. As a dad, I know this—you want to soak in every minute and revel in the joy, not live in anxiety and fear. Fortunately for our patients who use the techniques described in this book, relief is often just around the corner. Now, we are able to bring these same proven techniques to you. I wish you success in overcoming your anxiety problem. The peace you will feel will be well worth the effort.

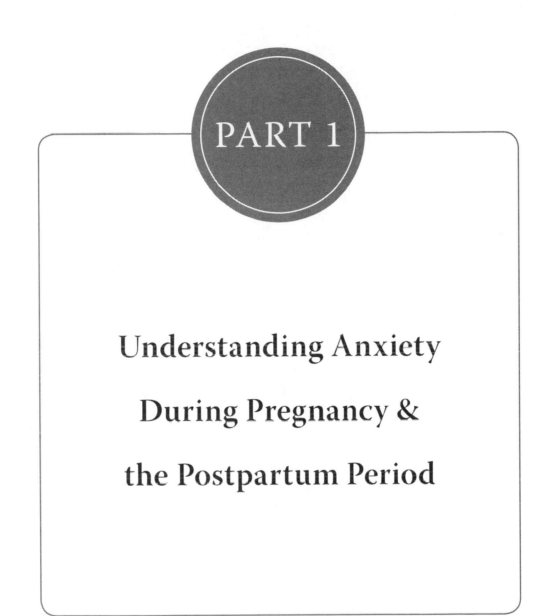

PART 1

Understanding Anxiety During Pregnancy & the Postpartum Period

CHAPTER 1

Understand Anxiety During Pregnancy & the Postpartum Period

You've no doubt heard about postpartum depression. If you have a television, you've probably seen at least one celebrity mom talking about her experience with depression after delivering her baby. But something you may not be aware of is how common anxiety is during and after pregnancy. Studies have found that anxiety disorders are actually *more* frequent than depression during pregnancy, and at least as common as depression during the postpartum period (Brockington, Macdonald, and Wainscott 2006), if not more so (Wenzel et al. 2005). Although you may not hear a lot about anxiety during pregnancy and the postpartum period, you are not alone in experiencing it—many, many women suffer from anxiety while pregnant or following the birth of a child.

Anxiety during and after pregnancy is only beginning to get the attention that it deserves. There is much left to discover, but we are finally recognizing anxiety in new moms and moms-to-be and appreciating its impact on both mother and child.

In this chapter we'll give you a brief overview of what is currently known about anxiety during pregnancy and in the postpartum period. You'll learn about how common anxiety problems really are, what makes you vulnerable to them, and the effects that untreated anxiety can have on you and your baby.

How Common Is Anxiety During Pregnancy and the Postpartum Phase?

Given that about one-third of women will suffer from an anxiety disorder at some point in their life (Kessler et al. 1994), maybe we shouldn't be surprised that anxiety is common among new moms and moms-to-be. In fact, some anxiety during pregnancy and early motherhood is universal—it would be unusual for you to *not* be anxious during this time. But, for many women, this normal anxiety can escalate and become an anxiety *disorder*—a term for anxiety that is severe enough to cause you great distress or interfere with your ability to function well at home or at work. Anxiety during and after pregnancy can range from normal worry and anticipation to severe, incapacitating fear.

Because this is a rapidly evolving field of study, reported rates of anxiety problems during pregnancy and the postpartum phase vary greatly. We do know that many women struggle with fear and worry during this time. Researchers note anywhere from 5 to 16 percent of women have an anxiety disorder during pregnancy or the postpartum period (Kelly, Zatzick, and Anders 2001; Wenzel et al. 2005). In addition, many more women experience symptoms of anxiety disorders that do not meet formal diagnostic criteria but nevertheless impair their ability to function. And this phenomenon is worldwide. Studies from countries as far away as Turkey, Brazil, Australia, and Nigeria have reported high rates of anxiety during pregnancy and the postpartum period and its negative effects (Sayil, Gure, and Ucanok 2007; Faisal-Cury and Menezes 2007; Grant, McMahon, and Austin 2008; Adewuya et al. 2006).

Exercise: Talk to Your Doctor

If you don't already have an upcoming checkup scheduled, call your obstetrician and schedule an appointment. Make notes beforehand regarding any important information or questions you have for your doctor. You can take along a copy of this book to share with your doctor and his or her staff, if you'd like. Tell them in detail how you are feeling—don't assume that they can guess. And don't be embarrassed. Remember—you are not alone! It may be hard for you to have this conversation, but know that you are doing what's best for you and for your baby.

Why Don't More People Talk About Anxiety During Pregnancy and the Postpartum Phase?

In the public eye, postpartum depression and its risks have overshadowed anxiety during pregnancy and the postpartum phase, but we hope that this is beginning to change. Those who suffer from anxiety know just how devastating its effects can be. However, at present, only about 20 percent of obstetrician-gynecologists (OB-GYNs) say that they routinely screen for anxiety during pregnancy (Coleman et al. 2008) and only about one-quarter of anxiety cases are recognized by their obstetricians (Smith et al. 2004; Coates, Schaefer, and Alexander 2004). As researchers continue to bring this important issue to the forefront, things will change. Until then, the message is clear: If you are a pregnant or new mom and you are struggling with anxiety, tell your obstetrician! Don't wait for someone to ask— too many women suffer in silence. Take an important first step on the road to recovery and let your doctor know that you are anxious.

What Is Known About Anxiety in New and Pregnant Moms?

The short answer? Not enough. Much more research is needed before we can truly understand the complex interplay of factors involved in producing this common problem. You might guess that hormonal influences play some role in the development of anxiety during this period. This is certainly the case, although direct relationships remain unclear. Several changes in the brain during pregnancy—such as alterations in certain neurotransmitter and neurohormone systems—may help to explain vulnerability to anxiety during and after pregnancy (Altemus et al. 2004). Ironically, though, some of the changes that occur during pregnancy, like increased oxytocin and prolactin, may contribute to *suppression* of the stress response (Altemus and Brogan 2004). These hormones can have calming effects and may actually *decrease* the brain's reactivity to stress. Despite those potentially protective effects, however, a large number of women still complain of anxiety during pregnancy. This paradox makes it difficult to fully understand the effects of pregnancy hormones on anxiety and makes it clear that hormones are not the only culprit. Unfortunately, the bottom line is that we simply don't yet know why some women develop anxiety symptoms in response to pregnancy while others do not.

The hormonal changes that occur during pregnancy, however, may help us to better understand why postpartum moms are at high risk for anxiety problems. The rapid changes that occur in brain neurochemistry during the transition from pregnancy to the postpartum period may lead to anxiety in susceptible women (Altemus et al. 2004). If the brain has difficulty compensating for this abrupt drop in pregnancy hormones and making subsequent adjustments in neurotransmitter systems, anxiety disorders may follow. For some women, the impact of this process may be buffered by breastfeeding, which makes the transition from pregnancy more gradual and protects against the drastic hormonal fluctuations that accompany the postpartum period. Indeed, researchers have found that breastfeeding women seem to have fewer anxiety symptoms than bottle-feeding moms do (Carter, Altemus, and Chrousos 2001; Mezzacappa et al. 2000). However, these effects are certainly not universal—in fact, breastfeeding itself can be a source of stress for some moms. We still have much to learn about the effects of pregnancy-related changes on anxiety during pregnancy and the postpartum period. Until we know more, women in these phases will

~ COMMON QUESTION ~

What might make me vulnerable to anxiety during pregnancy and the postpartum period?

One of the biggest factors to predict anxiety in new and pregnant moms is a history of anxiety (Breitkopf et al. 2006). Simply put, if you have had anxiety problems in the past, you may be vulnerable to relapse during pregnancy or the postpartum period. Other characteristics, like perfectionism, are also strongly related to anxiety during this time (Vliegen et al. 2006). For example, you may begin to buy into the supermom myth, believing that you should be perfect and able to do it all, and this may contribute to the development of anxiety and depression. Life experiences may further influence who develops anxiety and who does not. For instance, women who have had miscarriages in the past are at increased risk of experiencing persistent anxiety symptoms (Geller, Kerns, and Klier 2004); moms with high-risk pregnancies also tend to show high levels of anxiety during pregnancy (Brisch et al. 2005).

still be vulnerable to anxiety problems such as panic attacks, obsessions, compulsions, worry, and post-traumatic stress.

The Risks of Untreated Anxiety During Pregnancy and the Postpartum Period

Besides the discomfort that anxiety causes, there are several good reasons to pay attention to your anxiety during and after pregnancy. As we've said, it is normal to be anxious while pregnant or just after having a baby—motherhood practically guarantees some fear, anxiety, and worry. It just comes with the territory. However, severe, prolonged, or incapacitating anxiety can be harmful and should be addressed. Below, we've summarized some of the risks that untreated anxiety problems pose to both you and your baby.

Risks to You

Maybe the most consistent finding in the research literature is that clinically significant anxiety during pregnancy puts you at risk for postpartum depression (Heron et al. 2004; Austin, Tully, and Parker 2007). In fact, in some studies, women with anxiety during pregnancy were nearly three times more likely to experience symptoms of depression following the birth of their child (Sutter-Dallay et al. 2004). And, not surprisingly, anxiety during your pregnancy also puts you at risk for anxiety after delivery (Grant, McMahon, and Austin 2008). Women with anxiety have also been found to have more physical complaints during pregnancy (Kelly, Russo, and Katon 2001) and may be vulnerable to the development of post-traumatic stress reactions to childbirth (Keogh, Ayers, and Francis 2002).

Risks to Your Baby

Beyond the risks posed to you by an anxiety problem, it can also have potentially damaging effects on your baby. The first place you may find these effects is in the pregnancy and delivery itself. Though some studies have found no adverse neonatal outcomes (Dayan et al. 2006), other have found low APGAR scores in babies of moms with anxiety during pregnancy (Berle et al. 2005) and increased risk of preterm birth (Orr et al. 2007; Mancuso et al. 2004).

Babies of moms who suffer from anxiety during pregnancy have been found to have more difficulty in new situations (David et al. 2004) and behavioral and emotional problems in preschool years (O'Connor, Heron, and Glover 2002). In fact, the effects of anxiety during pregnancy have been found in kids up to age fifteen in areas such as attention and impulsivity (Van den Bergh et al. 2005). Maternal anxiety can also lead to "difficult" temperament in infants (Austin et al. 2005) and difficulty soothing (Coplan, O'Neil, and Arbeau 2005). As you can see, anxiety during pregnancy and the postpartum period seems to have lasting effects on children that may leave them vulnerable to behavioral or emotional problems down the road.

Next Steps

Having read the above information, you may be feeling even more anxious than you were before, but don't despair—the rest of this book is dedicated to helping you learn what you can do to overcome your anxiety and ensure a happy, healthy experience with motherhood. It is designed to help you beat your anxiety problems by learning strategies and skills that you can apply whenever anxiety strikes.

Now that you understand what may make you vulnerable to anxiety and the damage it can cause, you are ready to get to work. Begin now and put yourself on the path to a more peaceful pregnancy and relaxed start to motherhood.

Key Points

- Anxiety during pregnancy and after delivery is quite common.

- If you are anxious, it is important to share this with your obstetrician.

- Hormones may be partially responsible for anxiety during pregnancy and the postpartum period, but other factors likely play a role as well.

- Anxiety poses risks for mothers as well as potentially long-lasting negative effects on babies.

- You can use this book to develop a personalized plan to beat your anxiety.

CHAPTER 2

Learn About Treatment Options

If you're like most of the clients who come to our offices asking for help with their anxiety, your first question is "How can I feel better?" Decades ago, we wouldn't have had a good answer for you. Back then, anxiety problems were considered chronic and largely untreatable. If you suffered from anxiety, you could expect to either spend years on an analyst's couch recounting stories from your childhood or take habit-forming medications.

Fortunately, the past few decades have brought tremendous advances in the treatment of anxiety. Cutting-edge research and innovative clinical practice have opened the door to effective treatment, and the prognosis for anxiety problems is now excellent. There's now good reason to hope for swift, long-lasting improvement. These days, we actually have good answers to the question "How can I feel better?"

In this chapter, we'll describe the two most effective forms of anxiety treatment. First, we'll discuss a type of therapy known as cognitive behavioral therapy. You'll learn what cognitive behavioral therapy is and how it works. We'll also give you a brief overview of medication therapy, the other effective form of anxiety treatment. We'll then help you weigh the risks and benefits associated with these treatments and formulate a plan to talk with your doctor about your options.

Cognitive Behavioral Therapy

Cognitive behavioral therapy (CBT) is one of the most exciting advances in the treatment of anxiety over the last century. CBT is a form of psychotherapy that focuses on how two things—your thoughts and your behavior—affect your mood. The central philosophy behind CBT is that if you change how you think and act you can change how you feel.

The goal of CBT for anxiety is simple—a significant reduction of your anxiety problem. For example, let's suppose that as you approach your third trimester you have started having panic attacks. The goal in using CBT is to reduce or eliminate your panic attacks and help you restore a sense of calm to your life. Or, let's imagine that, since learning that you're pregnant, you've started worrying constantly and it's affecting your health and your relationships. In CBT, the goal is to help you decrease your worry and rid yourself of its harmful effects.

Does CBT Work?

We use CBT in our practices for two reasons. One is that the research on CBT is compelling. Study after study shows that it's a highly effective form of anxiety treatment (Chambless and Gillis 1993). The second reason is that we see the value of these techniques every day in our work.

For example, a client of ours named Jody came to therapy when she became pregnant with her first child. Though Jody was excited to become a mom, once she found out she was pregnant she started having intense feelings of anxiety and panic because of a long-standing phobia that she had never addressed: Jody was afraid of vomiting. Amazingly, she had somehow managed to avoid vomiting for the previous twenty years. Now, she was terrified she'd throw up due to morning sickness.

Fortunately, Jody sought help. With some persistence, courage, and hard work, Jody used the techniques described in this book, and in just a few weeks she conquered the fear that had plagued her for two decades and threatened to ruin her pregnancy. She was now able to enjoy her pregnancy experience and enter motherhood on a positive note.

Jody's experience is not uncommon. In fact, researchers have found that CBT is an effective form of treatment for every kind of anxiety problem (Chambless and Gillis 1993). Today, many experts consider CBT the gold standard of treatment of anxiety disorders. It's fast and effective, and you can easily apply the techniques on your own.

CBT in Pregnancy and the Postpartum Period

CBT has been well established as the psychological treatment of choice for anxiety, but studies are just emerging that show its effectiveness during pregnancy and the postpartum phase. Techniques like relaxation have been shown to significantly reduce anxiety during pregnancy (Teixeira et al. 2005). In one study CBT during pregnancy was found to significantly lower anxiety levels, and these gains were maintained through the postpartum period as well (Austin et al. 2008). Interestingly, in that study, giving women information about anxiety and depression and self-strategies to prevent and manage these problems, rather than formal cognitive behavioral therapy, was also found to be effective in reducing anxiety. Groundbreaking findings like these reinforce what we already know from our clinical practice: CBT is an effective strategy for reducing anxiety during pregnancy and the postpartum period. Whether you are working with a therapist or on your own, you can use the cognitive behavioral techniques in this book to address your anxiety, fear, and worry during and after pregnancy.

Pros and Cons of CBT

As effective as CBT is for anxiety, it's important for you to consider the pros and cons of any form of treatment before you make a decision on how to tackle your own anxiety problems. Let's take a look at some of the pros and cons of CBT.

Pros of CBT

- You won't have to take medication and expose yourself and your child to the risks of medication use during pregnancy and while nursing and recovering from the birth.

- You'll learn specific tools and techniques to manage your anxiety now and in the future.

- The rate of relapse for anxiety problems is often lower with CBT than it is with medication, so you'll be less likely to have recurring symptoms.

Cons of CBT

- CBT requires you to invest a significant amount of time and effort to overcome your anxiety problem.

- The exposure-based techniques used in CBT may temporarily increase your anxiety.

- You may have difficulty finding a trained CBT therapist.

This last con—finding a trained CBT therapist in your area—is unfortunately a common problem. However, one of the most exciting aspects of CBT is that, with a little guidance, you can apply these strategies on your own, so you might not need a therapist to help you. In the chapters ahead, you'll find step-by-step descriptions of effective techniques you can use to defeat your anxiety. Our goal in writing this book is to teach you how to use the tools of CBT to manage your own anxiety. Once you master the use of these tools, you can conquer your anxiety once and for all.

Exercise: Consider the Pros and Cons of CBT

Above, we've listed some common issues to consider as you decide how to tackle your anxiety problem. However, everyone's list of pros and cons will be different. Take out a sheet of paper and draw a line down the middle. On the left side, write "Pros of CBT" and on the right side write "Cons of CBT." On that sheet, make a list of your own pros and cons of using CBT to conquer your anxiety. Then take a look at your list. Which side wins? Does CBT come out on top? Or do the cons outweigh the pros? This list can help you think through your decision as you develop your plan to defeat your anxiety.

Medication Options

The other main type of treatment available for anxiety problems is medication. There are two main classes of medications for anxiety: antidepressants and antianxiety medication. If you're pregnant or nursing, medication can be a particularly frightening option. You've worked hard to avoid risks to your child and, understandably, you may worry that taking medication could harm your baby. Although it's true that medication is a potential risk, it is also an effective option for anxiety that is often used during pregnancy. We believe it's important for you to know the facts so that you can talk to your doctor and make an informed decision.

Antidepressants

The name of this class of medication can be a bit misleading. These drugs are called antidepressants because they were initially developed to treat depression. Since then, the antidepressants have been proven to be effective in treating other problems as well, including anxiety. The main type of antidepressant in use today is the selective serotonin reuptake inhibitor (SSRI), although serotonin-norepinephrine reuptake inhibitors (SNRIs) or tricyclic antidepressants can also be used. These medications usually take about two to four weeks to start working. They are generally well tolerated but can cause side effects early in treatment. It is important to be aware that antidepressants can actually *increase* feelings of anxiety and jitteriness in the first couple of weeks. If you decide to try medication, you may find some of the relaxation techniques in chapter 4 helpful during that initial period.

SSRIs include the following drugs:

- Citalopram (Celexa)

- Escitalopram (Lexapro)

- Fluoxetine (Prozac)

- Fluvoxamine (Luvox)

- Paroxetine (Paxil)

- Sertraline (Zoloft)

Anti-anxiety Medications

The other main class of anxiety medications are those known as anti-anxiety medications, which have two main types, benzodiazepines and azapirones. These medications help in treating the physical symptoms of anxiety.

Benzodiazepines

The benzodiazepines are a group of fast-acting anti-anxiety medications that are often used for short-term relief of anxiety symptoms. Some of the most commonly prescribed benzodiazepines include the following:

- Alprazolam (Xanax)
- Clonazepam (Klonopin)
- Lorazepam (Ativan)
- Diazepam (Valium)

Azapirones

Azapirones are similar to the SSRIs in that they seem to act on receptors for serotonin and may take two to four weeks to show an effect. Buspirone (BuSpar) is the azapirone most commonly used for anxiety.

When to Consider Medication

The decision to take psychiatric medication while you are pregnant or nursing can be a difficult one, but there are certainly times where the benefits of medication can outweigh the risks, such as in the case of severe anxiety, or if you are suffering from both anxiety and depression. In particular, you should consider taking medication if your anxiety problem is significant enough that it could harm you or your child.

How can you know if your anxiety problem is severe enough for you to consider medication? No one but you can truly answer that question—taking medication is a personal decision and every case is unique. We've noted some situations in the checklist exercise on the next page, however, in which you should consider medication. This list is nowhere near complete, but you can use these guidelines to help you make your choice (Nonacs et al. 2005).

> ### ~ COMMON QUESTION ~
> #### Can I use both medication and CBT to treat my anxiety?
>
> Absolutely. CBT and medication are often combined to treat anxiety problems. In addition, these two forms of therapy can complement each other effectively. Medication can be used to quickly reduce some of your anxiety symptoms while you are learning the skills and techniques of CBT to manage your fears over the long haul.

Medication Decision Checklist

The checklist summarizes the risk factors that might lead you to consider medication to treat your anxiety problem. Take a moment and check off any symptom you've had in the past two weeks.

Symptoms	Yes	No
Do you have thoughts of harming yourself or committing suicide?		
Have you experienced a lack of appetite leading to weight loss or inadequate weight gain during pregnancy?		
Does your anxiety problem significantly interfere with your ability to care for yourself or your baby?		
Have you had trouble complying with pre- or postnatal care recommendations?		
Do you use alcohol or other substances to manage your anxiety?		
Do you have symptoms that worry you or those who know you?		

If you checked yes for any of the symptoms above, make an appointment with your obstetrician or physician to discuss medication as an option to treat your anxiety. An open and honest discussion with your doctor can help you to determine, together, the best treatment options for you and your child.

Pros and Cons of Using Medication

Deciding whether to use medication to treat your anxiety problem can be difficult. Being pregnant or in the postpartum phase only complicates the decision. Again, as is the case with considering CBT for your anxiety, you may find it helpful to look at the pros and cons.

Pros of Medication

- It's an effective form of treatment for anxiety.
- It's readily available.
- With antidepressants, you can expect to see results within two to four weeks.
- The benzodiazepines relieve anxiety much quicker, usually within thirty minutes.
- If your anxiety is severe, medication may reduce it enough for you to effectively participate in CBT.

Cons of Medication

- If you're pregnant or breastfeeding, you'll expose your baby to medication.

- Once you stop taking medication, your symptoms could return.

- Benzodiazepines can be habit forming.

Exercise: Consider the Pros and Cons of Medication

Take a look at the list above and consider some of the pros and cons of using medication to manage your anxiety. Now take out another sheet of paper, draw a line down the middle and write "Pros" on the left and "Cons" on the right. Make a list of your own pros and cons of using medication. As you review your list, which side wins? Is considering medication a good idea for you or too much of a risk? This list can help you prepare to talk with your doctor about taking medication to treat your anxiety.

Talking with Your Doctor About Taking Medication

Now you know the basic medication classes used to treat anxiety, and you've considered the pros and cons of medication use during pregnancy and the postpartum period. If you are considering medication, the next step is to talk with your obstetrician. The information above is meant to arm you so you can make an informed choice. However, any medical decisions regarding your health and your baby's health should be made only after close consultation with your doctor, or with an appropriate psychiatrist or reproductive psychiatrist referred by your doctor. You can also turn to the resource list near the end of this book for ideas on where to find a qualified provider.

Here are some questions to ask your doctor when you discuss medication for the treatment of your anxiety:

- What are the risks of medication to me or my baby?

- Are there any other treatment options, such as CBT?

- What are the risks to me or my baby if my anxiety is left untreated?

- How do these risks compare with general rates of pregnancy complications or birth defects?

- Do I need to see a specialist, like a psychiatrist, to discuss medications?

- Will being pregnant affect the way my medications work?

Exercise: Talk About Medications with Your Obstetrician

If you've decided that medication is an option you want to consider, the next step is to have a frank discussion with your obstetrician. Take a moment and prepare before you meet with your doctor. You'll want to make sure you have a chance to ask all of your questions so you can be informed and aware of all the risks and benefits of medication. Take out a sheet of paper and make a list of questions before your meeting. You can use the questions above as a guide. Be sure to add any other questions you might have as well.

Next Steps

Now that you know the options available to treat anxiety, you're ready to work through the rest of this book. In the pages ahead, you'll find key cognitive behavioral techniques specifically designed to help you manage anxiety. If you feel that you also need a therapist to help you work through your anxiety, you can use the list of resources near the end of this book to find an appropriate provider.

Key Points

- Two effective methods are available to treat anxiety problems: cognitive behavioral therapy and medication.

- Cognitive behavioral therapy is an effective form of therapy that focuses on modifying the thoughts and behaviors that lead to your anxiety.

- Two main types of medication are used to treat anxiety: antidepressants and anti-anxiety medication.

- To decide what treatment is right for you, consider such factors as the severity of your anxiety, the availability of different types of treatment, your time and other constraints, and your tolerance for risk.

- A frank discussion with your obstetrician or psychiatrist can help you to decide which type of treatment is best for you.

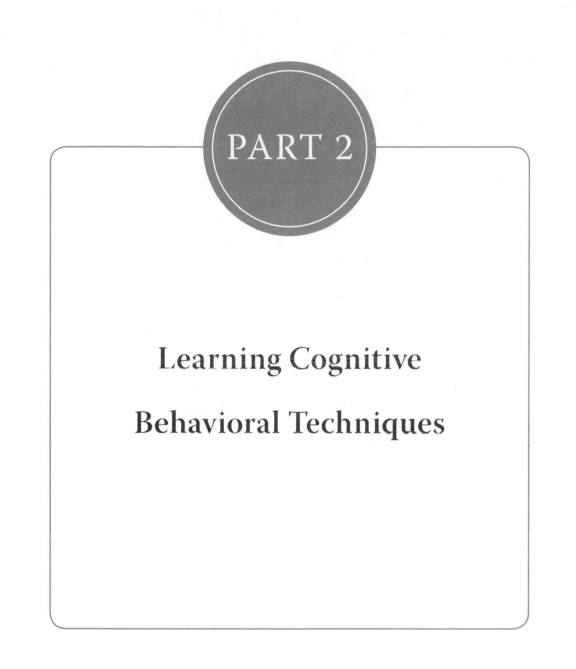

PART 2

Learning Cognitive

Behavioral Techniques

CHAPTER 3

Assess Your Anxiety Symptoms

Jane was enjoying one of the simple pleasures of parenthood: giving her three-month-old baby, Connor, a bath. After she placed Connor in the tub, Jane smiled and cooed at him as he gently kicked the soapy water. She took out a washcloth, squeezed some lavender-scented shampoo on it and started washing Connor's hair. Then suddenly—out of nowhere—a terrifying thought hit her: "What if I drown him?" Frantic, she quickly pulled Connor out of the bath, wrapped him in a towel, and drained the tub.

Maria was seven months pregnant when she awoke with a start in the middle of the night. She was sweating, her heart was pounding, and she felt gripped by intense fear. Her mind raced. "What's wrong with me? Oh my God, I'm having a heart attack!" She jumped out of bed and paced up and down the hall, her veins flooded with adrenaline. Minutes later, the feeling of terror started to fade. Still shaking, Maria climbed back into bed, wondering what had just happened to her.

Sara couldn't wait to have Taylor. She was so excited; the nine months seemed to fly by. However, shortly after her daughter was born, Sara's excitement turned to fear. Her biggest worry was sudden infant death syndrome (SIDS). She was terrified that her daughter would die in her sleep. To cope with this fear, Sara started a checking ritual. Several times a night, she went into Taylor's bedroom and checked her breathing. "Just one more breath," she told herself as she watched Taylor sleeping peacefully, "so I can make sure she's okay."

What do Jane, Maria, and Sara have in common? How can we explain their experiences? Though their symptoms are very different, all three are suffering from an anxiety problem. In this chapter, we'll describe the common types of anxiety problems that women experience as they become mothers. We'll also guide you through a self-assessment test so you can identify your own anxiety symptoms. Then, you'll use the information you gain from that assessment to help you locate the sections of this book that will be most helpful to you.

Common Anxiety Symptoms in New and Pregnant Moms

Anxiety symptoms are a common experience of both pregnant and postpartum women. If you had problems with anxiety before you became pregnant, these symptoms may worsen during pregnancy or after the birth. Even if you've never had trouble with anxiety before, as a pregnant or new mom you may be particularly vulnerable to certain kinds of anxiety. These include the following symptoms:

- Panic attacks
- Obsessions
- Compulsions
- Worry
- Post-traumatic stress symptoms

We'll describe each of these anxiety issues in more detail below.

Panic Attacks

A panic attack is a sudden, intense rush of fear that usually lasts for about ten to fifteen minutes. If you've ever had a panic attack, you probably felt like you were having a heart attack, going crazy, or about to die. Panic attacks are frightening, especially since they often seem to come out of nowhere. The good news is that, even though they can be terrifying, panic attacks are generally harmless. However, panic attacks can disrupt your life, especially if they happen frequently or if they cause you to avoid things, such as driving or being in crowded places.

Panic attacks are usually accompanied by intense physical symptoms that can include (American Psychiatric Association 2000) the following:

- Racing heart
- Lightheadedness or dizziness
- Numbness or tingling sensations in hands or feet
- Sweating
- Trembling
- Feeling short of breath
- Feeling of choking
- Chest pain or discomfort
- Nausea
- Fear of losing control or going crazy

- Fear of dying
- Chills or hot flashes

It is also common to develop *safety behaviors* in response to panic attacks. Safety behaviors are behavioral responses you use in order to cope when you feel panicky. They could be things like distracting yourself, carrying medication or a cell phone with you at all times, or only going to places you fear if someone accompanies you. Safety behaviors are often comforting in the moment, but in the long run they only make anxiety worse.

> ~ COMMON QUESTION ~
> ### What if I can't go anywhere without feeling anxious?
>
> Recurring panic attacks can result in *agoraphobia,* a condition in which a person avoids certain activities or places out of fear of having a panic attack. For example, you may avoid things like grocery shopping or going to the park with your child. Not everyone who suffers from panic attacks will develop agoraphobia. If you have agoraphobia in addition to your panic attacks, you'll benefit from the information in the rest of this book as well.

Obsessions

An obsession is an unwanted and intrusive thought, impulse, or image that causes distress. Though there are many types of obsessions, new moms commonly experience four main types of obsessions:

- Contamination
- Doubting
- Harming
- Sexual

Contamination Obsessions

When people think of obsessive-compulsive disorder (OCD), they usually think of contamination. Contamination is one of the most common fears in OCD. It's been dramatized in popular movies like *As Good as It Gets* and *The Aviator,* in which the main characters suffered from this disorder. As you might guess, "contamination OCD," the label for this type of OCD, consists of obsessive thoughts about getting contaminated in some way. For example, you might have obsessive thoughts about contracting a particular disease after touching a doorknob or using a public restroom. Or you might fear contamination from a harmful substance, such as mercury or lead. For instance, Cecilia was preoccupied with the idea that her young daughter, Ellie, might somehow become contaminated by lead. She began to fear lead contamination when their turn-of-the-century home was being renovated. Despite no evidence of the presence of lead in her home, Cecilia could not shake the idea that Ellie might get lead poisoning. She repeatedly sent samples of paint and water in for testing, stocked up on bottled water, and avoided touching the walls of her house. She began restricting her daughter to certain areas of her home and eventually even sent her to stay with her grandparents for fear that she would be harmed by contamination.

Doubting Obsessions

A doubting obsession is one where you're unsure about something and you feel compelled to get certainty about it. For example, when Jill's son, Evan, was born, the nurse put an ID bracelet on his wrist. Later that day, while they were still in the hospital, Jill noticed that she could read the ID number on Evan's bracelet both forward and backward. Unfortunately, each way produced a different number. Because of this numerical anomaly, Jill began to wonder if she had the right baby. The nurses at the hospital reassured her, but Jill still had doubts. Even after Jill took Evan home from the hospital, she didn't feel certain. Her doubts made her so anxious that she asked her husband and doctor repeatedly if Evan was really her child. Jill started checking a small mole on Evan's lower back dozens of times a day to confirm that it was him. She even thought about having DNA testing to make sure she had the right baby.

Harming Obsessions

Research shows that parenthood is a time when women—and men—are particularly vulnerable to developing harming obsessions (Abramowitz, Schwartz, and Moore 2003). In a harming obsession, the parent has unwanted thoughts of harm coming to his or her child. For example, you might have an obsessive thought that your child will get run over by a car or suffocate in his sleep. Actress Brooke Shields, who struggled with postpartum depression and anxiety, reported that she experienced a harming obsession in the form of an image of her baby flying across the room, hitting the wall, and sliding to the floor (Shields 2005). You might also have harming obsessions in which you fear directly causing harm to your child. For instance, you might have obsessions about harming your baby by drowning, stabbing, choking, throwing, hitting, or smothering him or her.

An important feature of these thoughts is that they are *ego-dystonic*. This means that the thoughts are inconsistent with your personality and violate your moral values and beliefs—in other words, you don't actually want or intend to act on them. Harming obsessions are distressing precisely because you wouldn't want any harm to come to your child.

~ COMMON QUESTION ~
Who *has* these kinds of thoughts?!

As upsetting as harming and sexual obsessions can be, researchers have shown that these types of thoughts are common. For example, some studies have found that 100 percent of new moms had intrusive thoughts of harm befalling their infant (Fairbrother and Woody 2008). In that same group, 50 percent of the moms also reported thoughts of intentionally harming their newborn either physically or sexually.

You've no doubt heard of high-profile cases where a mom actually does harm her children. These moms are usually suffering from other forms of mental illness, such as postpartum psychosis, not anxiety. However, if you find your harming or sexual thoughts pleasurable instead of distressing, if you have a history of violence or inappropriate sexual behavior, or if you feel you are in danger of acting on your thoughts, please consult with a medical or mental health professional immediately. You should also seek professional help right away if you are hearing voices, thinking people are against you or out to get you, or feeling uncontrollable anger (Baer 2001).

Sexual Obsessions

As the name suggests, sexual obsessions consist of thoughts or images of sexually molesting your child. With many moms, these unwanted, intrusive thoughts occur during close physical contact with their baby. For instance, you might experience these obsessions when you're diapering or bathing your child. Or you might have this type of thought during breastfeeding or physical play, such as tickling. Like harming obsessions, these thoughts are distressing precisely because you would never choose to act on them and they are in stark contrast with your personality and values.

Compulsions

Compulsions or rituals are repetitive behaviors designed to ward off disaster or reduce distress. Compulsions usually occur in response to an obsession. For example, if you have contamination fears, you might find that you wash your hands excessively. Or, if you have doubting obsessions, you might feel compelled to engage in habitual checking.

Common compulsions include the following:

- Checking

- Washing

- Avoidance

- Reassurance seeking

- Mental

Checking Compulsions

Checking rituals are extremely common. They consist of repeatedly checking specific things such as locks or electrical appliances. Checking compulsions can occur with any obsessions but they are most common with doubting obsessions. For example, if you suffer from doubts about whether you have locked the door or turned off the stove, you might repeatedly check to quell your fears. And, ironically, despite your repeated checking, you might still feel strong doubts and intense anxiety.

Washing Compulsions

Washing is another common compulsion. Compulsive washing can include things such as hand washing, showering, or cleaning. Washing usually occurs in response to contamination fears. For instance, if you are afraid you will get ill from germs or bacteria, you might wash your hands excessively.

Avoidance Compulsions

Avoidance—staying away from things that trigger your obsessive thoughts—is often overlooked as a compulsion. However, it is a common way that people with obsessions cope with their disturbing thoughts. Avoidance is a typical behavior in people with harming obsessions. For example, if you have fears of hurting your new baby, you might avoid holding her or being alone with her.

Reassurance-Seeking Compulsions

This compulsion consists of repeatedly seeking reassurance from other people or information sources. For example, if you have fears about your baby's health, you might repeatedly ask your significant other if the baby looks ill. Or, if you have sexual obsessions, you might scour the Internet for information on sexual predators in an effort to reassure yourself that you would not act on these thoughts.

Mental Compulsions

Many people are unaware that compulsions can be mental as well. A mental compulsion is something you think repeatedly in response to an obsession. For example, if you experience harming obsessions, you might think, "I would never hurt my child," or repeat silent prayers to yourself whenever you notice a harming thought.

Worry

We define worry as catastrophic thinking about the future. For example, you might have thoughts such as "What if I can't breastfeed?" or "What if my marriage falls apart?" These thoughts both fit the definition of worry because they involve two types of thinking:

- Catastrophic thinking—thoughts about a worst-case scenario.

- Future-oriented thoughts—worries about the future, or about something that hasn't happened yet. You can usually tell that you're thinking about the future when you have a "what if" thought.

Of course, everyone worries at times. However, if your tendency to worry goes unchecked, you might also suffer physical symptoms (American Psychiatric Association 2000) such as the following:

- Restlessness

- Fatigue

- Difficulty concentrating

- Irritability

- Muscle tension

- Insomnia

Marcy, who was six months pregnant with her first child, worried night and day that her child might have a birth defect. Despite reassuring prenatal test results, Marcy could not stop thinking about the possibility that her baby might have a congenital defect. She lay awake at night, tired but unable to sleep, with "what if" thoughts racing through her mind. It was difficult for her to concentrate on much else and she often found herself worrying and pacing in the kitchen at three o'clock in the morning or searching the Internet for information.

As is the case with those experiencing other anxiety problems, people who worry often have behaviors that they perform in an attempt to decrease anxiety. These are called *worry behaviors*. Worry behaviors don't actually have a real effect on the outcome; they just make the person feel better temporarily. Marcy's habit of searching the Internet for information on birth defects is a good illustration of a worry behavior. Other examples are superstitions, reassurance seeking, and avoidance.

Post-traumatic Stress

Symptoms of post-traumatic stress are often associated with combat veterans returning from war. However, post-traumatic stress can affect anyone. In fact, post-traumatic stress is more common in women than in men and can occur after many types of traumatic experiences, like domestic violence, rape, childhood sexual abuse, labor and delivery, or any experience where a person feels intense terror, horror, or helplessness (American Psychiatric Association 2000).

Reexperiencing the trauma is one of the main symptoms of post-traumatic stress. This usually occurs in one or more of the following ways:

- Intrusive thoughts or images

- Nightmares

- *Flashbacks,* or acting or feeling as if the event is happening again

In addition to reexperiencing the trauma, you might find that you avoid people, places, or situations that remind you of the trauma. Many people who suffer from post-traumatic stress also experience symptoms of chronic nervous system arousal, such as difficulty sleeping, irritability or anger, or difficulty concentrating.

June had a history of childhood sexual abuse but felt, after therapy, that she had finally put this terrible experience behind her. She was in a loving marriage, overjoyed at the prospect of becoming a mom, and eagerly planning for her new arrival. She weathered the first two trimesters well but, in her third trimester, the discomfort and physical sensations associated with carrying a growing baby began triggering memories of the past abuse. She found herself thinking often of the perpetrator and had nightmares, and she began avoiding visits to her obstetrician. The excitement she had felt in the early months was gone and she now avoided talking about the baby and resisted any attempts by her husband or doctor to discuss a plan for labor and delivery.

Common Anxiety Problems in Moms	
Anxiety Problem	**Symptoms**
Panic attacks	• Sudden, intense rushes of anxiety • Avoidance of activities or places (agoraphobia)
Obsessions	• Unwanted, intrusive thoughts, images, or impulses that cause distress • May be contamination, doubting, harming, sexual, or other types
Compulsions	• Repetitive rituals designed to reduce anxiety or prevent something bad from happening • May include washing, checking, reassurance-seeking
Worry	• Uncontrollable, catastrophic thoughts about the future • Physical symptoms such as headaches or fatigue
Post-traumatic stress	• Recurrent intrusive thoughts, images, or nightmares about a traumatic event in the past • Avoidance of people, places, or other things related to trauma • Symptoms of chronic arousal, such as insomnia or feeling edgy or jumpy

What Are Your Anxiety Symptoms?

Now that you know the different types of anxiety that women often experience while pregnant or following the birth of a child, it is time to take a close look at whether you are having any of these symptoms.

Exercise: Assess Your Anxiety Symptoms

Use the worksheet below to identify the type of anxiety problem you may have. Answer yes to any question if you've experienced the symptom for much of the time over the past two weeks. Keep in mind that anxiety disorders tend to cluster together, so, if you've been feeling anxious, you may have experienced many different anxiety symptoms, and you may find that you check off several boxes.

Panic Attacks and Agoraphobia

1. I experience sudden, intense rushes of anxiety that appear to come "out of the blue." ☐ Yes ☐ No

2. During these attacks, I fear having a heart attack, going crazy, fainting, losing control, or some other catastrophic event. ☐ Yes ☐ No

3. I avoid certain activities or places, such as driving or elevators, because I'm afraid I'll have a panic attack. ☐ Yes ☐ No

Obsessions

1. I experience unwanted, intrusive thoughts, impulses, or images that I can't seem to get rid of. ☐ Yes ☐ No

2. These thoughts cause me distress. ☐ Yes ☐ No

Compulsions

1. I engage in repetitive behaviors such as hand washing or checking and I find these behaviors very difficult to stop. ☐ Yes ☐ No

2. I use these behaviors to lessen my anxiety or to prevent something bad from happening. ☐ Yes ☐ No

Worry

1. I worry excessively about different aspects of my life, such as finances, work, or relationships. ☐ Yes ☐ No

2. I find it difficult to control my worry. ☐ Yes ☐ No

3. My worry causes physical symptoms such as headaches, muscle tension, or fatigue. ☐ Yes ☐ No

Post-traumatic Stress

1. I've experienced one or more traumatic events in the past during which I felt intense fear or helplessness. ☐ Yes ☐ No

2. I have intrusive thoughts, images, or recurring nightmares about this event. ☐ Yes ☐ No

3. I avoid places, people, activities, or other things that remind me of the traumatic event. ☐ Yes ☐ No

4. I have symptoms of chronic arousal, such as irritability or jumpiness, or I have difficulty concentrating. ☐ Yes ☐ No

Keep in mind that these questions are designed to give you a feel for the kind of anxiety you're experiencing and guide you to the sections of this book that will be the most helpful to you. They're not meant to be a substitute for a diagnostic evaluation by a mental health professional. If you find that your anxiety problems are significantly interfering with your life, please contact a mental health professional who is trained and experienced in the treatment of anxiety disorders.

Exercise: Your Anxiety Checklist

Use the checklist below to note any anxiety problems that you identified in the self-assessment exercise.

Anxiety Problem	Yes	No
Panic attacks		
Obsessions		
Compulsions		
Worry		
Post-traumatic stress		

Does answering yes in the exercise above mean you have an anxiety disorder? Not necessarily. Feeling anxious at times is universal—who hasn't had a rush of anxiety when they suddenly realized they forgot something important or had a close call while driving? Anxiety disorders are diagnosed when symptoms are severe enough to cause interference in your ability to function in the important areas of life, such as work, relationships, or school.

This book is designed to help you with *any* troubling anxiety symptoms you experience, whether you have an anxiety disorder or not. Even if your symptoms aren't severe enough to qualify as a disorder, you can still use the techniques described in this book to feel better. In our view, you don't need to have a diagnosable disorder to reduce your anxiety symptoms.

Next Steps

Now that you know what kind of anxiety you're experiencing, you're ready to work on overcoming it. At this point, you can go on to chapter 4 and start using the techniques that will help you manage your anxiety effectively.

Once you master the techniques in part 2, you can jump right to the chapters in part 3 that specifically address your symptoms. In the chart below, we've listed the chapters in this book that target the specific problems pregnant or new moms are likely to experience.

Anxiety Problem	Chapter
Panic attacks	8
Obsessions	9
Compulsions	9
Worry	10
Post-traumatic stress	11

Key Points

↬ If you are a new mom or mom-to-be, your existing anxiety symptoms may worsen or you may be more vulnerable to developing certain types of anxiety problems. These include panic attacks, obsessions, compulsions, worry, and post-traumatic stress symptoms.

↬ The self-assessment exercise in this chapter will help you to identify which anxiety symptoms you are experiencing.

↬ Once you determine which anxiety problems are troubling you, you'll be ready to use the rest of this book. Start by learning the techniques described in part 2, and then select the chapters in part 3 that address your specific issues.

CHAPTER 4

Develop Relaxation Skills

Having a baby, whether it's your first or your fifth, is one of the most exciting events you can experience. It's also one of the most stressful. With all that having a child demands of you, from doctor visits to sleepless nights to picking out a name, it probably seems like you barely have time to breathe. Plus, as if the demands of motherhood aren't taxing enough, they can also make anxiety problems such as panic attacks or worry even worse.

Fortunately, there's hope. By mastering some straightforward and effective relaxation techniques, you can learn to relax and enjoy this wonderful time in your life instead of letting stress and anxiety spoil it. In this chapter, we'll describe three key techniques for achieving a state of deep relaxation: *diaphragmatic breathing, progressive muscle relaxation,* and *guided imagery.* These techniques are essential building blocks in the process of managing stress and anxiety.

Before You Begin

Before you start practicing the techniques described in this chapter, you need to know the following three important things about relaxation:

1. Relaxation is a skill.

2. Being a relaxed mom has real benefits.

3. There are ways to get the most from your relaxation practice.

Relaxation Is a Skill

Before you try these techniques, keep in mind that the ability to relax is a skill. And, like with any skill, you must practice it consistently to master it. You might find that thinking of relaxation as a skill is a bit unusual at first. After all, most of us think of relaxing as something passive, like sunning at the beach. Though lounging in the sun can certainly be relaxing, the benefits are usually temporary. The well-being you feel often fades along with your tan.

By using the techniques in this chapter, you'll be taking a proactive, long-term approach to relaxation instead. You'll be carving out time each day to experience deep relaxation. Not only will you feel great in the moment, but over time you'll also notice a host of other benefits that will improve your overall health and well-being while keeping your anxiety and stress at bay.

The Benefits of Being a Relaxed Mom

Some of the benefits you can expect from practicing relaxation on a daily basis include the following:

- Physical: slower heart rate, lower blood pressure, more energy

- Mental: greater concentration, sharper focus, improved memory

- Emotional: less anxiety and irritability, more positive mood

- Behavioral: better sleep, increased productivity

- Overall health: fewer headaches, decreased pain, less stomach upset

In short, by mastering the relaxation techniques in this chapter, you'll sleep better, feel better, be healthier, and experience less pain.

~ COMMON QUESTION ~
Can I use these techniques to help with the pain of labor and delivery?

Definitely! Pain can follow a vicious circle. When we experience something painful, we usually tense up. For example, think of how you feel the moment before you get a shot. If you're like most people, you tense up a bit. Unfortunately, this muscle tension only increases pain.

Facing a painful experience while physically relaxed, on the other hand, makes it hurt less. Lamaze, one of the most popular labor-pain management techniques, includes breathing and distraction techniques to reduce physical tension and lessen pain. The breathing, relaxation, and imagery techniques described in this chapter will also help you to decrease anxiety and physical tension. With practice, you can use these techniques not only to feel more relaxed on a daily basis but also to make labor and delivery a less stressful and painful experience.

Getting the Most from Your Practice: Keys to Successful Relaxation

Before you start learning to relax, take note of the following tips, which will help you get the most out of your practice:

1. Allow for about twenty minutes of practice time.

2. Choose a quiet spot where you won't be disturbed.

3. Turn off your phone and dim the lights.

4. Sit or lie down in a comfortable position.

5. Remove shoes and glasses. Loosen any tight clothing.

6. Try not to fall asleep during practice. The goal of relaxation practice is to experience and remember what being relaxed feels like so you can bring back the same feeling in stressful situations. If you fall asleep, you'll miss the experience.

7. Remember, repetition is the key. Commit to practicing daily.

Relaxation Technique No. 1: Diaphragmatic Breathing

Molly has suffered from panic attacks and worry ever since she was a teenager. Now in her early thirties and pregnant for the first time, Molly is noticing that her panic attacks have become increasingly frequent. Recently, she noticed that whenever she enters a situation that makes her anxious, such as driving in heavy traffic or riding the subway, her breathing becomes shallow and quick and she feels a bit lightheaded and dizzy. In other words, when Molly becomes anxious she *hyperventilates*.

Hyperventilation simply means breathing faster and deeper than necessary. When you hyperventilate, you take in more oxygen than your body needs. This causes the level of carbon dioxide in your blood to fall and leads to unpleasant—but harmless—physical symptoms such as lightheadedness, dry mouth, fatigue, numbness or tingling, and shortness of breath.

Hyperventilation is often the result of *chest breathing*. Chest breathing means moving the location of your breath from your stomach up into your chest. For many people, like Molly, this shift in breathing occurs when they feel stressed or anxious. The physical changes of pregnancy—namely a baby constricting the movement of your diaphragm—can also lead to chest breathing and hyperventilation.

When you're calm and relaxed, on the other hand, you breathe in a slow, rhythmic way, your stomach gently expanding and contracting, just like a balloon slowly fills with and releases air. Breathing this way is known as *diaphragmatic breathing*. To see a great example of diaphragmatic breathing, watch a sleeping baby. Notice how her stomach slowly and easily moves in and out with each breath.

Exercise: How Do You Breathe?

Check your own breathing. Place one hand on your chest and the other on your belly button and take a few normal breaths. Which hand moves? The more the hand on your chest moves, the more you are breathing from your chest and the more likely you are to experience symptoms associated with hyperventilation.

Instructions for Diaphragmatic Breathing

Diaphragmatic breathing counteracts the unpleasant effects of chest breathing and hyperventilation and creates a state of calm and well-being. To practice diaphragmatic breathing, follow the steps below:

1. Sit or lie down in a comfortable position. If you are more than twenty weeks pregnant, or if lying flat is uncomfortable for you, lie on your left side or sit in a semireclined position.

2. Let go and relax any tense muscles.

3. Turn your attention to your breathing and take a few deep, slow breaths through your nose. Focus on your breathing and feel yourself starting to relax.

4. Place one hand on your chest and the other on your abdomen, right above your belly button.

5. Try to move the location of your breathing from your chest to your abdomen. Your chest should remain still. Your stomach should expand and contract easily and effortlessly with each breath.

6. Once you're breathing into your diaphragm, try to slow your breathing down by counting to three as you breathe in and again as you breathe out.

7. When you're breathing at a pace of three counts in and three counts out and you are breathing into your diaphragm, continue for approximately ten minutes.

8. Focus on the feelings of relaxation deep breathing creates. Enjoy.

Practicing Diaphragmatic Breathing

Diaphragmatic breathing usually takes about a week of daily practice to master. Aim to practice for about ten minutes a day. On the relaxation skills form below, you can record your practice sessions. Be sure to make plenty of copies so you can record the dates you practiced and rate how relaxed you felt before and after you practiced. You can rate your relaxation on a scale of 1 to 100, with 1 being extremely tense and 100 being completely relaxed. Keep trying until you can consistently achieve a state of deep relaxation using this technique, scoring between 80 and 100 on the relaxation scale after practicing.

~ COMMON QUESTION ~

Can I practice diaphragmatic breathing if I'm still pregnant?

Sure. However, diaphragmatic breathing while you're pregnant can be difficult, especially as your pregnancy progresses to the later stages. If you find it difficult to move your stomach up and down while breathing because of your pregnancy, you can focus on slowing your breathing instead. Review steps six through eight and practice slowing down your breathing to three counts in and three counts out.

Relaxation Skills Practice Record

0—10—20—30—40—50—60—70—80—90—100
Very Tense   Average   Very Relaxed

Date of Practice	How Relaxed Did I Feel Before I Practiced? (0 to 100)	How Relaxed Did I Feel After I Practiced? (0 to 100)

On the next page, we've included a copy of Denise's practice record as an example. Denise was about seven months pregnant when she began practicing diaphragmatic breathing. As you can see, through daily practice, Denise began to feel more relaxed during the day and developed her ability to relax deeply at will using this technique. However, during her first session, she didn't feel more relaxed afterward, because she actually hyperventilated and felt lightheaded. This experience is common to people who are beginning to practice diaphragmatic breathing. With a few modifications in her technique, though, Denise was able to enjoy the full benefits of relaxation practice.

Denise's Relaxation Skills Practice Record

0—10—20—30—40—50—60—70—80—90—100
Very Tense   Average   Very Relaxed

Date of Practice	How Relaxed Did I Feel Before I Practiced? (0 to 100)	How Relaxed Did I Feel After I Practiced? (0 to 100)
04/24/07	5	5
04/25/07	10	25
04/26/07	10	75
04/27/07	15	75
04/28/07	15	85
04/29/07	20	85

If You Have Trouble

If you are having any difficulty relaxing using this technique, try the following tips:

- Try placing a book on your stomach. Practice moving it up and down with each breath.

- Since this technique involves slowing your breathing down, you might feel the need to take a deep breath, yawn, or sigh. Try to resist this urge and aim to keep your breathing steady and slow instead. Though you may feel momentarily uncomfortable stifling the desire to take in more air, resisting this urge will maximize your feeling of relaxation.

- You might feel a bit lightheaded at times during your practice, especially at first. This is normal. It's a sign that you're breathing too deep and hyperventilating a little bit. If this happens, try slowing down your exhalations and taking in less air when you inhale.

Relaxation Technique No. 2: Progressive Muscle Relaxation

Progressive Muscle Relaxation (PMR) (Jacobson 1929) is another effective technique you can use to achieve a state of deep relaxation. This technique is based on the idea that it's impossible to be both relaxed and tense at the same time. PMR teaches you how to voluntarily create a state of deep relaxation so you can drive away feelings of tension, anxiety, and stress.

Exercise: Where Are You Tense?

Everyone tenses different muscles when stressed. Before you begin PMR, identify where you are holding your stress by mentally scanning your body. Using the checklist below, identify the key spots that feel tense. Pay particular attention to these areas as you practice PMR.

☐ Arms   ☐ Back

☐ Legs   ☐ Face

☐ Neck   ☐ Chest

☐ Lips   ☐ Shoulders

Instructions for PMR

The steps below take you through the process of tensing and then relaxing specific muscle groups. For each step, tense the muscle group for ten seconds and then relax that muscle group for twenty seconds. As you move through the steps, try to tense only the specific muscle group in each step. Once you've relaxed a muscle group, keep it relaxed for the rest of the practice session. If, because of pregnancy or childbirth or another other issue, you find any step difficult or painful, just skip it:

1. Sit comfortably in a chair. With palms facing down, make a fist with each hand and pull your wrists up toward your bicep, creating tension your forearms. Then release the tension and let your forearms and hands completely relax.

2. Next, pull your upper arms toward your sides, tensing your biceps. Keep your forearms relaxed. Now release your arms, letting them hang loosely and relax.

3. Now pull your toes upward toward your knees, flexing your feet. Feel the tension in your calves. Then let your feet gently release back to the floor, and relax your calf muscles.

4. Gently pull your knees together and lift your legs until your thighs feel tense. Now rest your legs and relax.

5. If you are able, gently pull your stomach in toward your back, tightening your stomach muscles. Now release the tension and relax.

6. Take a deep breath to tense your chest and hold it for about five seconds. Release the air slowly and relax.

7. Lift your shoulders up toward your ears, creating tension in your shoulders and neck. Let your shoulders gently drop and release all the tension.

8. Now gently press your head back, tensing the muscles in your neck. Then let go and relax your neck completely.

9. Press your lips tightly together, without clenching your teeth or tensing your jaw. Then let your mouth relax, letting go of any tension.

10. Next, close your eyes tightly, creating tension around your eyes. Then release and relax, feeling the tension drain away.

11. Now, pull your eyebrows down, trying to get them to meet in the middle. Feel the tension in your lower forehead. Then let your forehead relax.

12. Raise your eyebrows as high as possible, wrinkling your forehead. Now relax those same muscles and notice the feeling of relaxation this brings.

13. Now relax your entire body completely and breathe slowly for several minutes, saying "Relax" to yourself on each exhalation. Focus on releasing any remaining tension in your body, and enjoy the feeling of deep relaxation.

It typically takes about twenty to thirty minutes to complete a session of PMR. It can help to create a recording of the steps above to guide you during practice. Record yourself talking through the steps in a calm, soothing voice, and allow yourself plenty of time to tense and relax each muscle group.

Practicing PMR

PMR usually takes about two weeks of daily practice to master. Use the Relaxation Skills Practice Record to track your practice, rating your level of relaxation before and after practice on a scale of 1 to 100. Over time, as you become more skilled at PMR, you should see both numbers rise. This means you're experiencing an overall reduction in tension as well as becoming deeply relaxed during your practice. When you consistently score between 80 and 100 after you practice, you've mastered PMR.

If You Have Trouble

If you are having difficulty practicing PMR, try the following tips:

- PMR can be challenging, especially if you tend to tense your muscles when you're feeling stressed. Give yourself plenty of time to master this skill. With practice, you'll find that you can relax quickly and easily.

- PMR shouldn't hurt. Resist overtensing your muscles. If you find that tensing any of your muscles causes pain or cramping, try tensing in a gentler way.

- Ironically, trying to relax can sometimes cause you to feel anxious. This is known as *relaxation-induced anxiety* (Brown, O'Leary, and Barlow 2001). If this happens to you, continue your practice—the anxiety will most likely disappear after several practice sessions—or you can try another technique listed in this chapter.

Relaxation Technique No. 3: Guided Imagery

Becoming a mom is like leaping into the "great unknown." It's hard to know exactly what to expect. Will your child be a good sleeper, or will she be fussy and colicky? When will she walk? What kind of a mom will you be? How will having a baby affect your marriage?

Unfortunately, our brains don't like great unknowns—so our imagination tends to fill them in for us instead. If you're feeling anxious about being a mom, chances are your mind is filling in the future with images of disaster. For example, you might see yourself trapped in your home all day with a screaming baby. Or you might picture a never-ending parade of pesky in-laws traipsing through your house. Perhaps you imagine yourself up all night, exhausted, trying to calm a colicky newborn.

Guided imagery helps counter those upsetting images, using your mind's eye to calm you instead of frighten you. In the same way that imagining disaster creates a state of anxiety, picturing a serene, relaxing scene can instill a sense of calm and peace.

Instructions for Guided Imagery

The guided imagery scene in this chapter is from our book *10 Simple Solutions to Worry* (Gyoerkoe and Wiegartz 2006). To practice guided imagery, follow the steps below:

1. Lie down in a comfortable position. Remember, if you are more than twenty weeks pregnant you can lie on your left side or sit in a semireclined position.

2. Slow your breathing down.

3. Scan your body for tension and relax any tight muscles.

4. Continue breathing calmly and slowly as you vividly picture the scene (see Guided Imagery Scene, below). When you're finished, sit quietly for several minutes with your eyes closed and enjoy feeling deeply relaxed.

To make your practice more effective, you can use a tape recorder to record the script below in a calm, soft voice, allowing plenty of time to imagine each part. Then you can use the recording to direct your visualization during your imagery practice. If you plan to use imagery during labor and delivery, you can even take the recording along with you to the hospital.

Guided Imagery Scene

Picture yourself walking along the beach. The sun is shining high in the blue sky. It's warm and comfortable and you feel the salty breezes cooling your skin. The water is a deep blue. Waves gently roll in. As you stroll, feeling the sand between your toes, you leave your worries far behind. You feel the warm sun on your skin and it calms you. Along the way, you come to a comfortable, quiet spot and choose to lie down.

You stretch out on a blanket and listen to the waves coming in to the shore. Your breathing starts to move with the rhythm of the waves. The sun, shining overhead, continues to warm your skin. You focus on the warmth on your feet, feeling them becoming comfortably warm and heavy. Your breathing becomes deeper and slower and the warmth of the sun spreads up your legs to your calves, and then to your thighs and hips. Both of your legs are now pleasantly warm and heavy and relaxed. You notice the sounds of the waves gently rolling in and out, in and out, further soothing you.

Your breathing is deep and slow now and you feel calm and relaxed. The gentle radiance of the sun now spreads from your legs up into your abdomen. You feel the muscles of your stomach relaxing with the warmth, becoming smooth, still, and relaxed. Your skin feels warm as your stomach rises up and down, in time with the waves.

The warmth of the sun continues to reach throughout your body, moving up from your stomach and filling your chest. You feel a light glow in your chest, filling you with relaxation and peace. Your legs, stomach, and chest feel warm, heavy, and relaxed. You breathe with ease now, only feeling the warmth that is filling you.

Now, the focus of the sun's warmth moves to your fingertips and starts to relax them. That feeling moves through your hands and up into your forearms and biceps. Your arms get heavy, the muscles relaxing deeply as the warmth of the sun moves through them. Your breathing slows a little more as you sink even further into relaxation.

The sun moves the relaxing warmth up into your shoulders and neck. You feel them ease and drop slightly as you allow yourself to relax under the warm sun. You notice how warm, heavy, and relaxed your muscles feel, from your toes to your shoulders, all brought to a state of deep relaxation by the warm sun.

The relaxation moves throughout the rest of your body, up into your neck and face. You feel these muscles loosen, your face becoming very smooth, open, and calm. The sun gently warms your face, soothing away any tension. You feel very peaceful now, as peaceful as you've ever felt. You are deeply relaxed.

Breathe easily now and just enjoy the feeling of deep relaxation. Notice how warm and heavy you feel, how perfectly calm and relaxed you are at this moment. Bask in the sun, feeling the golden rays covering your skin, bringing soothing warmth to you, making you feel completely calm. You are fully relaxed.

Exercise: Create Your Own Guided Imagery Scene

Maybe the last time you were at the beach, you got a severe sunburn or stepped on a jellyfish. Maybe you prefer hiking. If, for whatever reason, you don't find the scene above relaxing, you can simply create your own. The only rule is that it be relaxing to you. To make your own script, simply do the following:

1. Pick a place that you find relaxing.

2. Describe that scene in detail, using all five senses.

3. Work from your feet up through your body to your neck, shoulders, and face.

4. Relax and enjoy.

Practicing Guided Imagery

Guided imagery can take one to two weeks to master. As is the case with the other techniques presented in this chapter, you'll know you've mastered guided imagery when you consistently score between 80 and 100 on the relaxation scale after you've practiced imagining the scene. You can use the Relaxation Skills Practice Record to track your level of relaxation before and after you practice.

If You Have Trouble

If you are having difficulty practicing guided imagery, try the following tips:

- Visualization—like all relaxation techniques—is a skill that improves with practice. If you find it difficult to imagine the scene above, stay with it. Your ability to imagine will improve over time.

- You might find that other thoughts enter your mind during guided imagery. If this happens, simply let them pass through your mind, and then return your focus to the guided imagery scene.

Next Steps

In this chapter, you have learned three effective ways of achieving a state of deep relaxation. Later in this book, you will learn how these techniques can also be used for specific anxiety symptoms, particularly panic attacks, worry, and symptoms of post-traumatic stress.

Which relaxation technique should you use? Once you've practiced all three relaxation techniques in this chapter, you can use the one that works best for you. Or, if you're struggling with a particular symptom, you can use the technique that's best suited for that symptom. In the chart below, we've matched relaxation techniques with symptoms of anxiety and stress you might experience.

Anxiety Symptom	Relaxation Technique
Lightheadedness, dizziness, fatigue, dry mouth, numbness, or tingling	Diaphragmatic breathing
Muscle tension, headaches, neck pain, or back pain	Progressive muscle relaxation
Images of catastrophe popping up in your mind	Guided imagery

Key Points

- Regular relaxation practice has excellent health benefits for new and expectant moms.

- Learning to relax is a skill that takes regular practice in order for you to master it and receive the full benefits.

- There are three main techniques you can use to achieve a state of deep relaxation: diaphragmatic breathing, progressive muscle relaxation, and guided imagery.

- Diaphragmatic breathing involves breathing slowly with your diaphragm. Progressive muscle relaxation consists of systematically tensing and relaxing specific muscle groups. In guided imagery, you imagine a relaxing scene, such as soaking up sun at the beach, letting the warmth deeply relax you.

- Remember: practice, practice, practice!

CHAPTER 5

Modify Anxious Thoughts

"I can't understand it," Jennifer said tearfully during a therapy session. "This is supposed to be one of the best times of my life, but every moment is filled with fear. My mind races all day long. What if I have a miscarriage? What if I'm a terrible mom? What if I don't have a "maternal instinct"? What if my son gets picked on? What if we get divorced and our baby grows up without a dad? That's all I think about and it's driving me crazy. I want to enjoy this time, but I can't. I feel miserable."

As Jennifer describes her worries, you can see the direct link between thinking upsetting thoughts and feeling anxious: Jennifer feels anxious because her mind is flooded with negative thoughts. In this chapter, you'll learn more about the connection between negative thinking and anxiety. You'll also see how these negative thoughts can be distorted—how we often fool ourselves when we're anxious. And, most important, you'll learn specific strategies to combat your anxious thinking.

Your Thoughts and Anxiety

Your thoughts have a powerful impact on how you feel. This connection between your thoughts and feelings is the basis for a type of treatment known as cognitive therapy. Cognitive therapy is based on the simple yet powerful idea that your thoughts affect your moods and that, by changing your thinking, you can change how you feel (Burns 1999). Decades of research has shown that cognitive therapy is a highly effective way to alleviate anxiety.

To understand the impact of your thoughts on how you feel, first think back to a time when you felt excitement and joy about becoming a parent. What was going through your mind at the time? Record these thoughts in the space below:

_____

_____

_____

As you wrote in the space above, you might have thought about the wonderful parts of parenting, such as seeing your baby smile for the first time or snuggling with her for a nap. Perhaps you looked to the future and thought about teaching your daughter how to ride a bike or accompanying your son on his first day of school.

Now, think about a time when you felt anxious, stressed, and overwhelmed about raising a child. What was going through your mind then? Record your thoughts below:

_____

_____

_____

As you review these thoughts, notice how they've turned toward the "dark side" of parenthood. Perhaps you wrote down thoughts focused on the challenges of parenting, like sleepless nights, temper tantrums, endless diaper changes, or money problems. Or maybe you came up with other worries and fears, like the health of your unborn child or the challenges of juggling work and motherhood.

As you can see from these examples, how you think largely determines how you feel. If you're thinking about something in a negative light, you'll probably feel upset or anxious. Similarly, when you feel relaxed, you see things in a more realistic, optimistic way.

In this chapter, you'll learn three key steps to turning your thinking around and taking control of your anxiety:

1. Identify your anxious thoughts.

2. Label any distortions in your thinking.

3. Replace your anxious thoughts with more accurate, realistic thinking.

Identify Your Anxious Thoughts

The first step toward changing your thinking is to identify the negative thoughts you have when you're feeling upset or anxious. To help you zero in on those thoughts, it's important to find out what kind of events or situations trigger your negative thinking. These triggers represent the anxiety-producing situations you face regularly as a new mom or mom-to-be.

Exercise: List Your Activating Events

Think back over the past week or so. When did you feel especially anxious? What time of day was it? What was happening at the time? Where were you? Who were you with? What were you doing? Answering these questions will help you figure out what events trigger your negative feelings. List five of your activating events on the lines below:

1. _____

2. _____

3. _____

4. _____

5. _____

Once you've identified the situations that trigger your anxiety, choose one situation from the list above. Now ask yourself what you were thinking at the time. What was going through your mind? What kind of thoughts do you recall having? How about images or daydreams?

Now use the chart below to start working on these anxious thoughts. Briefly describe the situation that triggered your negative thinking, note how you felt, and jot down your negative thoughts.

Cognitive Therapy Worksheet: Step One		
Situation	**Feelings**	**Anxious Thoughts**

For example, Joan went out to dinner with her husband one night during her second trimester. While they were enjoying their meal, Joan noticed a mom in the restaurant trying to calm a crying newborn. Joan began to feel anxious and depressed. She recorded these thoughts on her Cognitive Therapy Worksheet: Step One.

Joan's Cognitive Therapy Worksheet: Step One		
Situation	**Feelings**	**Anxious Thoughts**
Seeing a stressed-looking mom trying in vain to calm a crying infant	Anxious Depressed	That's going to be me. We'll probably have a colicky baby who cries all the time. I won't be able to enjoy my child. We'll all be miserable.

As you can see, watching a stressed-out mom struggling to calm her crying child was an activating event for Joan. At that moment, Joan's thoughts turned black, like storm clouds sweeping across the horizon. She began to think about her future as a mom in a highly negative way. The result was that Joan felt anxious and depressed.

Label Your Cognitive Distortions

Now that you've identified the thoughts that make you feel anxious, let's take a closer look at them. When you're feeling anxious or upset, your thoughts are often *distorted*—in other words, unrealistic or illogical in some way.

Below, we've listed some of the most common ways thinking can get distorted, along with some examples of each type of distortion. Take a look at this list and consider your own thoughts. Do any of these distortions sound familiar?

All-or-Nothing Thinking

All-or-nothing thinking means seeing the world in extreme categories. By viewing the world in this way, you ignore the subtleties in favor of a rigid, black-and-white take on things.

Examples of all-or-nothing thinking include the following:

- "I'm a bad mother."

- "I didn't follow all of the doctor's instructions, so I'm a failure."

- "I have to be a perfect mom."

Overgeneralization

When you're engaged in the cognitive distortion of overgeneralizing, it means you're making global inferences based on a few experiences. One clue that you're overgeneralizing is the presence of the word "always" or "never" in your thoughts.

Here are a few examples of overgeneralizing:

- "My child cries all the time."

- "My newborn never sleeps."

- "I never get to have an adult conversation with my husband anymore."

> ### ~ COMMON QUESTION ~
> #### Does everyone have distorted thoughts?
>
> Absolutely. Even when we're not feeling anxious or depressed, we all engage in distorted thinking at times. However, when our mood sours or we feel anxious, distorted thoughts take over and make it difficult to think in a clear, realistic way. Cognitive therapy is about restoring your ability to see things in a reasonable, balanced light and improving your mood in the process.

Mental Filtering

Mental filtering occurs when you focus exclusively on the negatives and blot out the positives. You'll know you're using a mental filter when you catch yourself focusing on one negative aspect of a situation at the expense of everything else. For example, you might think only of the sleepless nights during the first few months of having a child—while overlooking the joys of being a mom—and allow that to blacken your view of parenthood.

Below we've listed some examples of mental filtering:

- "Motherhood is all work."

- "All our baby does is cry and poop."

- "Our baby cried all through dinner and totally ruined the night."

Discounting the Positives

Having a new baby is full of wonderful moments and difficult challenges. Unfortunately, if your thinking is affected by this distortion, you won't register the wonderful moments in your consciousness. Especially in the beginning, the rewards of parenting may be a bit limited. Your baby probably won't even smile at you until a month or two after she's born! You may have to move mountains of coal to find a few small diamonds. If you discount the positives, you'll insist that the good things you and your baby do "don't count" and instead dwell exclusively on the negatives.

Here are a few examples of discounting the positives:

- "I don't deserve credit for my hard work—it's what a mom should do."

- "Everyone is supposed to follow doctor's instructions while pregnant, so I didn't do anything special by taking care of myself and my baby."

- "So what if my baby took a nap? He cried the rest of the day."

Overestimating the Threat

As the name suggests, overestimating the threat means that you've taken something that may involve a slight risk and made it seem threatening and dangerous. With the sometimes-frightening information available to you as a new mom or mom-to-be, you might find this a particularly common distortion.

Examples of overestimating the threat include the following:

- Fearing standard vaccines even though the rate of complications is low

- Thinking that your baby will be kidnapped from the hospital nursery

- Being afraid to stand near a microwave while pregnant

Catastrophic Thinking

When you're engaged in catastrophic thinking, you take minor setbacks and view them as horrible, awful, and unbearable. In fact, those are key words to watch out for when you're on the lookout for catastrophic thinking. If you notice words such as "awful," "horrible," or "terrible" crossing your mind in reaction to minor difficulties, you may be engaged in catastrophic thinking.

Examples of catastrophic thinking include the following:

- "If my baby doesn't feed well right away, that will be horrible."

- "It's awful to let my baby cry at all."

- "It'll be terrible if I don't lose this baby weight."

Fortune Telling

One constant in parenting is change. Babies and children develop and grow so quickly that it's often hard to predict what tomorrow will be like, much less next month. When you distort your thoughts with fortune telling, you disregard the fact that you can't predict the future, and you make what may seem like iron-clad guarantees about what will happen next.

Here are some examples of fortune telling:

- "With my luck, we'll have a fussy, colicky baby."

- "I know my husband won't be any help once our child is born."

- "I'm never going to get any sleep."

"Should" Statements

"Should" statements are rigid rules about how you, your baby, and the world "should" be. If you direct a "should" toward yourself, you'll feel guilty and inadequate. In contrast, "should" statements directed toward other people make you feel frustrated, helpless, and angry.

Examples of "should" statements include the following:

- "I should always have loving, warm feelings toward my child."

- "I should immediately know what my baby wants when she cries."

- "My husband should know that I need help around the house."

"What if" Thinking

"What if" thinking means you scare yourself by asking "What if?" about bad things that might happen in the future. "What if" thinking is one of the most common distortions in anxiety. Chances are that, if you're feeling worried or anxious, this distortion is one of the culprits.

Examples of "what if" thinking include the following:

- "What if my son doesn't develop at the 'proper' rate?"

- "What if I accidentally drop my baby?"

- "What if I can't handle labor and delivery?"

Discounting Your Coping Skills

When you're feeling anxious, you're really telling yourself two things. The first is that something bad is about to happen. The second is that you can't handle whatever disaster you think is going to strike; you're telling yourself that you can't cope with difficulties, challenges, or setbacks.

Below, we've listed some common ways people discount their ability to cope:

- "I couldn't handle it."

- "I can't stand it."

- "I don't handle stress or challenges well."

One of our clients, an expectant mother named Margaret, started experiencing panic attacks during the first few months of her pregnancy. Although she was excited about having a child, when she felt panicked her thoughts became more pessimistic and negative. One night, when she was feeling especially anxious and panicky, she grabbed a pen and paper and wrote down the thought "I've made a mistake." What distortions do you see in this thought? As Margaret looked through the list of cognitive distortions, she saw that she was distorting her thoughts with all-or-nothing thinking, fortune telling, mental filtering, and discounting the positive.

Cognitive Distortions

1. **All-or-nothing thinking:** You force experiences into one of two extreme, black-or-white categories, such as good or bad, or perfect or completely wrong.

2. **Overgeneralization:** You make broad, global inferences based on just a few events. If the words "always" and "never" appear in your vocabulary, you may be overgeneralizing.

3. **Mental filtering:** You focus on one or a few negative aspects of a situation and allow them to spoil the whole thing.

4. **Discounting the positives:** You insist that the good things you or others do "don't count."

5. **Overestimating the threat:** You take a situation that involves slight or no risk and make it seem threatening and dangerous.

6. **Catastrophic thinking:** You view a minor setback as horrible, awful, or terrible.

7. **Fortune telling:** You make iron-clad predictions about dire things happening in the future.

8. **Should statements:** You apply rigid, absolute rules to yourself and others about how things "should" and "shouldn't" be.

9. **"What if" thinking:** You ask "What if?" about bad things happening in the future.

10. **Discounting your coping skills:** You tell yourself that you can't cope with problems or difficulties.

Exercise: Label Your Cognitive Distortions

Now that you're familiar with the different types of cognitive distortions, let's see if you can find any distortions in your own negative thoughts. Choose a thought from the Cognitive Therapy Worksheet you completed previously and then take a look at the list of cognitive distortions. What distortions do you see in your thought? Keep in mind that one thought can contain many different distortions.

In the worksheet below, jot down the situation, feelings, and thoughts from the worksheet you completed earlier. Then, using the list of cognitive distortions above, see what distortions you can find in your thoughts.

Cognitive Therapy Worksheet: Step Two			
Situation	**Feelings**	**Anxious Thoughts**	**Cognitive Distortions**

Let's also take a look at the thoughts Joan recorded while she was out to dinner with her husband and see what distortions she was able to find.

Joan's Cognitive Therapy Worksheet: Step Two			
Situation	**Feelings**	**Anxious Thoughts**	**Cognitive Distortions**
Seeing a stressed-looking mom trying in vain to calm a crying infant	Anxious Depressed Angry	That's going to be me.	Fortune telling
		We'll probably have a colicky baby who cries all the time.	Fortune telling, all-or-nothing thinking, discounting the positives, mental filter
		I won't be able to enjoy my child.	Fortune telling, discounting coping skills, discounting the positives
		We'll all be miserable	All-or-nothing thinking, mental filtering, discounting the positives, discounting coping skills, catastrophic thinking

How to Change Your Thinking

Now that you've learned to identify your negative thoughts and know the common ways that your thoughts can get distorted, it's time to learn some powerful methods to turn your thinking around. The techniques listed below are key strategies for thinking in a more balanced, realistic way. Consider them part of your tool kit for alleviating anxiety. These ideas and techniques are based on the work of leading cognitive therapists such as Judith Beck (1995), David Burns (1999), and Robert Leahy (2003).

Examine the Evidence

When we have negative thoughts, we often accept them as gospel without examining them. One way to challenge your negative thoughts is to critically examine the evidence for and against them. You can do this by asking yourself the following questions about your negative thoughts:

- "What's the evidence that supports my negative thought?"
- "What's the evidence against my negative thought?"
- "Which side is more convincing?"
- "What should I do now?"

Generate Alternatives

When you feel anxious, you mentally lock in on the worst-case scenario. For example, if you feel a twinge in your abdomen, you might think, "I'm having a miscarriage." Or, if your husband is quiet and withdrawn one night, you tell yourself, "He is not interested in me anymore." An effective way to counter this worst-case scenario tendency is to generate alternative explanations.

Ask yourself the following questions in response to your negative thoughts:

- "What's the worst-case scenario?"

- "What's the best-case scenario?"

- "What's the most likely scenario?"

- "What are at least three other possibilities?"

Anticatastrophic Thinking

When you feel anxious, your mind fills with catastrophic thoughts and images. One antidote to this tendency is to ask yourself a series of questions designed to "decatastrophize" your thinking:

- "What is the worst that could happen?"

- "How likely is it that the worst would actually happen?"

- "What could I do to cope if it did occur?"

- "How often have I been right in the past when I predicted catastrophes?"

Double Standard

We're often much more critical and more unrealistic toward ourselves than we are toward other people. When we are challenging a negative thought, it can be helpful to think of how we would respond to someone else who was in the same situation. This can allow you to be more objective, rational, and compassionate. For example, let's say you are feeling self-conscious about the weight you've gained during pregnancy. You tell yourself, "I'm so huge and repulsive right now. I can't bear to face anyone," and you decide that you don't want to go out with your friends.

Now ask yourself what you would say to a friend in the same situation. You'd probably be much more realistic, understanding, and caring. You might tell your friend, "It's okay. You're pregnant— you're supposed to gain weight. We don't want you to be perfect. We just want your company." This more-realistic mindset can serve as powerful ammunition against your own negative thoughts.

Image Substitution

When you're feeling anxious, terrible images of the future flood your mind. For example, if you are worried about the stress of becoming a parent, you might picture yourself up at four in the morning frantically trying to calm a screaming baby, exhausted, and up to your ears in diapers.

When you look into the future, however, you are imagining something that hasn't happened yet. Things can—and often do—turn out very different from the way we envision them. When you are playing horror scenes in your mind, remember that you do have a choice about what you imagine. The only thing you accomplish by imagining the worst in the future is to make yourself miserable in the present. How about a more pleasant, enjoyable scene instead? Perhaps you could see yourself gently cuddling your sleeping baby as you relax in a rocking chair. Or maybe you could picture yourself holding your baby's hand as he walks for the first time. Maybe you could imagine giving your daughter a warm bath as she happily splashes in the tub.

The next time you catch yourself picturing negative images, try countering them with a more positive scene instead.

Conduct an Experiment

Another way to challenge a negative thought is to simply test it out to see if it's true. For instance, you may feel lonely and isolated during the first few months with your new baby because you spend most of the time feeding, burping, and changing diapers. You'd love nothing more than to have lunch with one of your friends like you used to do. But, when pick up the phone to invite a friend to lunch, you think, "No one wants to have lunch with an exhausted mom and her screaming baby." So, you decide not to call and put the phone back down. You end up feeling even more alone.

How can you test out this thought to see if it's true? It's simple. Set up an experiment by calling several of your friends and asking them to lunch. That way, you can see if your negative thought is true—that no one wants to have lunch with you—or if you have been simply jumping to conclusions.

When challenging your negative or anxious thinking, ask yourself if you can conduct an experiment to see if your thoughts are actually true.

Talk to Other Moms

Being a mom can be an isolating experience, especially when your child is still an infant. The rigors of parenting often pull you away from the support of family and close friends. As a result, you can lose sense of what is "normal." It can help to check out some of your negative thoughts with your friends. Ask them if they have experienced the kinds of thoughts or feelings that you are having and how things ultimately turned out for them.

Caution: Choose carefully when deciding whom you'll survey. You'll get the most accurate responses from friends who have a baby close to yours in age. Those who have never had a child might not provide you with an accurate picture. And, for those with older kids, time has a way of making the past look rosier than it actually was—they might be the ones who say, "Jake slept through the night right away! It was a miracle!" Their skewed perspective might validate your fears and lead you to feel even worse. Instead, consider asking other moms in the same position as yours, or trusted professionals such as your pediatrician, for more accurate information.

Let's take a look at how Joan used these strategies to turn her thinking around—and change how she felt.

Joan's Cognitive Therapy Worksheet: Step Three					
Situation	Feelings	Anxious Thoughts	Cognitive Distortions	Coping Responses	Techniques
Seeing a stressed-looking mom trying in vain to calm a crying infant	Anxious Depressed Angry	That's going to be me	Fortune telling	Having a baby is challenging but it also has great rewards.	Examine the evidence
		We'll probably have a colicky baby who cries all the time	Fortune telling, all-or-nothing, discounting the positives, mental filter	Who knows? Maybe we'll have a great sleeper. I can cope with it once it happens.	Generate alternatives
		I won't be able to enjoy my child	Fortune telling, discounting coping skills, discounting the positives	Most likely, there will be a mix of both fun times and challenging times.	Anti-catastrophic thinking
		We'll all be miserable	All-or-nothing, mental filtering, discounting the positives, discounting coping skills, catastrophic thinking	Parenting is tough at times, but I doubt we'll be miserable all the time. Besides, I'm really looking forward to snuggling with my baby!	Double standard, image substitution

As you can see from Joan's worksheet, she used a variety of different techniques to defeat her negative thoughts. Now it's your turn. Take your negative thoughts you identified earlier and put them in the worksheet on the next page. Then use the techniques listed above to generate rational responses that accurately and believably dispute your negative thinking.

Cognitive Therapy Worksheet: Step Three

Situation	Feelings	Anxious Thoughts	Cognitive Distortions	Coping Responses	Techniques

If You Have Trouble

Identifying and modifying your negative thoughts are challenging skills to learn. It's normal to struggle at first. Here are some common difficulties that people face, and ways to overcome them.

Difficulty Identifying Negative Thoughts

Sometimes it's tough to figure out what you're thinking. You might say, "I'm not thinking anything. I just feel anxious." Keep in mind that, when you feel anxious, there's usually a negative thought lurking somewhere in your mind. It just might take some work to lure it out. If you're having difficulty identifying your negative thoughts, try the following:

- Take a guess about what might be going through your mind. Sometimes even a guess can provide the key to finding your negative thoughts.

- Consider times in the past when you felt the same way. What was going through your mind then? The same thoughts might be causing trouble again.

- Look for images as well as thoughts. Instead of thinking an actual thought, such as "I'll be up all night and never get any sleep again," you might be *picturing* yourself exhausted and up all night tending to a crying baby.

Difficulty Challenging Your Thought

Challenging and changing your thinking is often the hardest step. If you're having difficulty, keep in mind that persistence often pays off. Stick with it and be stubborn! You might have to struggle with a particularly tricky thought for a while until you finally crack it. Also, remember that it often takes multiple techniques to defeat a thought. If one of the strategies we listed above doesn't work, drop it and move on to another one.

If You Don't Feel Any Better

When you've successfully replaced a distorted negative thought with a more realistic, balanced response, you'll likely experience immediate relief. If you've completed the entire Cognitive Therapy Worksheet and you don't feel any better, there are probably two reasons:

- Your response isn't convincing. In other words, you don't really believe it. Telling yourself something you don't really think is true probably won't help much. Try to create a coping response that is based in fact so you can't help but believe it is true.

- You have overlooked an important negative thought. Go back and review your negative thoughts again. Did you catch them all on paper? Or are there some that you have missed? If you find one or more that you have overlooked, jot them down, identify the distortions, and then use the techniques described above to create a credible, effective coping response.

Next Steps

Practice completing an entire Cognitive Therapy Worksheet each day. Plan to spend about ten minutes jotting down your negative thoughts, identifying the distortions, and generating coping responses. If you get stuck on a thought, you can come back to it later. Often, you'll find that you have a fresh perspective when you return to a thought after taking a break from it. Once you feel comfortable identifying your anxious thoughts and generating effective coping responses, you should experience a noticeable change in how you feel. In part 3 of this book, you'll learn how you can apply this skill for specific anxiety symptoms, like worry, panic, and post-traumatic stress.

Key Points

- Remember, if you're feeling anxious, you're probably thinking anxious thoughts. Identify those anxious thoughts by writing them down on a blank Cognitive Therapy Worksheet.

- Once you've written your thoughts down, review the list of cognitive distortions and identify the distortions in your thoughts.

- Use the cognitive techniques listed in this chapter to replace your negative thoughts with more realistic coping responses.

- Be sure to write your responses down so you can review them in the future when you feel upset.

CHAPTER 6

Prepare to Confront Your Fears

Take a moment and think back to something you used to fear. Maybe you were afraid of the dark when you were a child, or dogs used to terrify you. Perhaps you were afraid of swimming or riding a bike. Now think for a minute—how did you overcome your fear? You probably overcame that fear by gradually and persistently confronting it. Maybe you started by playing with a puppy or dipping your toe in a wading pool and worked your way up from there. You were afraid, but you did it!

It sounds too easy, but it's true—one of the most effective ways for you to conquer your anxiety is simply to face it. Directly confronting your fears is known as *exposure therapy* or *exposure and response prevention* (ERP). Of course, directly confronting the things you fear—whether they are situations, thoughts, images or physical sensations—is not easy. You'll feel anxious at first. However, through repeated exposure, you'll learn that you can comfortably face these situations, fears, or worries. Exposure has been extensively studied and found to be a highly effective form of treatment for a variety of anxiety symptoms, including panic attacks, obsessions, compulsions, worry, and post-traumatic stress.

Response prevention is another effective way to overcome anxiety and is a key part of using exposure to decrease your fears. Response prevention is a strategy for letting go of the behaviors and avoidance that contribute to anxiety. This means that you identify any unhealthy strategies you use to cope with anxiety, such as checking, reassurance seeking, or avoidance, and eliminate them.

In this chapter, we'll describe exposure and response prevention as a way to reduce or eliminate your fears. Specifically, you'll learn the following:

- How exposure works and why it works so well

- How to use response prevention to make exposure even more effective

- How three different exposure techniques can help you overcome your fears

We've also included more specific applications of exposure and response prevention therapy to problems such as panic attacks, obsessive-compulsive symptoms, worry, and post-traumatic stress in part 3 of this book.

Habituation: How Exposure Works

Before you use exposure to overcome your fears, it's important to understand how and why exposure works. Research shows that if you engage in focused and repeated exposure to a thought or situation, your anxiety will decrease over time (Foa and Kozak 1986). This process is called *habituation*. It is our body's natural way of adjusting to repeated or prolonged contact with an object or situation.

For instance, think back to the first time you put on a watch or your wedding ring. For a while you were continually aware of the fact that you were wearing it. You may have even caught yourself adjusting the watch band or sliding the ring on and off your finger. This constant readjustment prolonged your awareness of its presence. But, once you left it alone, over time your body began to habituate to this new object, and now you barely know it's there. Believe it or not, the same process of habituation occurs with things you fear.

For example, Sandy felt anxious prior to her annual gynecological exam for as long as she could remember. She would put off making the appointments until her yearly exams became more like her "every-three-yearly" exams. For days and even weeks before, she would become anxious, imagining the discomfort and embarrassment she would experience. Sometimes she would cancel at the last minute, which only made her more anxious about the next appointment. When she became pregnant, she thought there was no way she would be able to manage the anxiety around all those required visits to the obstetrician.

But an amazing thing happened. Now that Sandy had to go in for these exams, she found that with each visit she became more and more comfortable. She faithfully kept to the exam schedule her doctor recommended, and her anxiety decreased with each completed appointment. In other words, now that she could no longer avoid her fears, her anxiety decreased—and eventually disappeared completely.

> ### ~ COMMON QUESTION ~
> #### What Should I Expect During Exposure?
> The overall effect of exposure will be a long-lasting decrease in anxiety, but you may find that initially your anxiety is higher than normal. This is expected and, in fact, your anxiety *needs* to be of at least moderate intensity during the exposure period in order for the exercise to be effective—consider this anxiety an investment in your calm future. As you confront your fears, you can expect to feel temporarily more anxious, but, if you stick with it, you should soon start to see positive results and reduced anxiety.

Response Prevention: The Key to Successful Exposure

When you are using exposure to lessen your fear, it's critical that you prevent rituals, safety or worry behaviors, and other unhealthy and ineffective coping strategies. For exposure therapy to work, you need to be anxious during the exposures and stick with it until you experience habituation. Anything that reduces your anxiety should be eliminated, because it can undermine your exposure efforts.

Look closely at your current coping strategies. Does your action actually address the problem you face or does it just make you *feel* better? If it is the latter, then it has to go! For instance, Julie feared that her son would die in his sleep. She would toss and turn at night, preoccupied with images of her son lying dead in his bed. As a result, she would check on him many times during the night to reassure herself that he was still breathing. This behavior temporarily lessened her anxiety but didn't change the end result—Julie's son survived the night because he was healthy and because it is rare for children to die in their sleep, not due to his mom's constant checking. In order for Julie to truly overcome her fear, she would need to stop compulsively checking on her son at night.

Common Types of Unhealthy Coping Behaviors

There are literally endless unhealthy ways of coping with anxiety, fears, and worries. We've listed a few of the more common ones below. As you read, see if you can identify any that you use. Remember, these coping strategies only *seem* like your friend—in reality they hold you hostage, making you believe that you need them in order to decrease your anxiety or to prevent negative outcomes.

Superstitions

These behaviors, based on unrealistic beliefs, are attempts to prevent your fears from coming true. By performing these behaviors, you convince yourself that you've decreased or eliminated the risk you faced. Practically speaking, however, these behaviors have no real impact on whether the outcome you fear will actually occur, and—worse yet—they may even lead you to worry *more*. For example, Sarah refuses to wear black during her pregnancy and she never discusses her baby in the future tense. Sarah believes that both of these behaviors reduce the chances of a miscarriage or stillbirth. They make Sarah temporarily feel better, but in actuality they have no effect on her pregnancy outcome.

Record any superstitious behaviors you may engage in below:

_____

_____

_____

Checking

As the name suggests, this type of behavior involves repeatedly checking to lessen your anxiety. For instance, Isabella has two young children and relies on checking the carbon monoxide detectors in her home several times a day whenever her fear of carbon monoxide poisoning strikes. Can you think of anything you do that may be considered a checking behavior? If so, write it down:

_____

_____

_____

Repeating

With *repeating*, you do something over and over in response to a worry or fear. It might mean reiterating a statement numerous times or repeating an action several times. For example, Ann is pregnant and worries about accidentally misleading her obstetrician during checkups. She fears giving the wrong information about things like how frequently the baby has been moving or whether she has experienced any unusual physical sensations. Ann deals with this worry by repeating herself excessively during visits and calling to "clarify" afterward to ensure she didn't accidentally mislead the doctor.

Can you think of times you excessively repeat statements or actions in order to lower your anxiety? If so, list them below:

_____

_____

_____

Reassurance Seeking

The essence of reassurance seeking is the attempt to eliminate doubt. You might ask for reassurance from friends or family members. You might consult experts, like doctors, for reassurance. Or you might compulsively search the Internet, books, or other sources of information. However you go about it, the goal is to find a guarantee that your fear won't come true. For example, Deirdre was unable to nurse her baby due to her financial need to return to work soon after delivery and her job, which did not lend itself to convenient pumping of breast milk. As a result, she worried constantly about her baby's health, convinced that she had doomed him to a frail and sickly life. She regularly searched the Internet for reassurance that formula-fed babies could also be healthy. Sometimes she felt convinced, after hours of searching, that her son would be fine. Other times, she still felt anxious and would repeatedly quiz her doctor, her friends, and her family to reassure herself. Unfortunately, the comfort she received was always short lived. Whenever her son developed a sniffle, or whenever an article on the merits of breastfeeding caught her eye, Deirdre began her search for certainty all over again.

Below, write down any ways that you excessively seek reassurance:

_____

_____

_____

Avoidance

The belief behind avoidance is that if you stay away from your fears, they won't come true. One of Lupe's biggest fears was that she wouldn't be able to handle labor and delivery. She feared that, when the time came, the pain would be so great and the experience so overwhelming that it would cause her to panic and have a meltdown in the delivery room. As a result, she avoided thinking about labor and delivery at all. She skipped over those chapters in her pregnancy book, changed the topic whenever it came up, and refused to sign up for the childbirth preparation class at her local hospital. In the short term, her strategy worked because she felt less anxious when focusing on the fun things like buying baby clothes, decorating the nursery, and registering for baby gifts. But, of course, there's a negative consequence to her avoidance. By ignoring this necessary stage of pregnancy, she denied herself information that might have actually decreased her anxiety and helped her have a more positive experience in the delivery room.

Can you think of any thoughts or situations you avoid due to anxiety? List them below:

_____

_____

_____

Why You Should Eliminate Avoidance and Unhealthy Coping Behaviors

Here's a question to ask yourself: Why would you continue these behaviors, when they don't actually influence the outcome of events? The most likely reason is because they bring you temporary relief from your anxiety. In other words, after completing them, you feel less anxious. The problem is, however, that the fear inevitably returns. And when that happens, you'll feel compelled to perform the behavior all over again. The result is a vicious circle. Because these actions neither solve the problem nor eliminate your worry, you must repeat them each time you feel anxious. And, in fact, not only must you repeat them whenever you get anxious but they also tend to lose their potency over time and you'll find that you need to do them more and more to get the same effect.

These behaviors also convince you that your actions prevent disaster. It's a compelling argument. Julie checks on her son several times a night. And each morning he wakes up full of smiles and ready for breakfast. Julie concludes that her checking has kept him safe. But why is he really still alive? Is it because of her checking? Or is it because the event she fears—her son dying in his sleep—is extremely unlikely to happen? By performing these behaviors, you never get to learn that the absence of disaster is not dependent on your actions.

Another reason you might continue these worry behaviors is your distorted perception of the consequences of not engaging in the behaviors. One of Jan's rituals was to completely avoid all foods that might be bad to eat during pregnancy, because she worried about the effects of these foods on the health of her baby. Despite her doctor's reassurance that it would be okay to eat fish occasionally or to have caffeine on a limited basis, she refused to indulge herself. She ate only organic products and carefully evaluated her daily nutritional intake for fear that if she strayed from this formula something would go wrong with her pregnancy. As a result, eating became a chore and she constantly felt tense because "but what if I don't and something goes wrong" kept ringing in her ears. It's that fear that bullies you into performing unnecessary behaviors each time you worry.

The next time you find yourself anxious and tempted to give in to your usual ineffective coping strategies, try something different—refuse to do anything! Your anxiety may rise at first, but stick with it. Before long, you'll feel your anxiety subsiding and you'll have taken an important step toward beating your fears once and for all!

How to Use Exposure to Conquer Anxiety

Now that you understand how avoidance and unhealthy coping behaviors maintain your anxiety and you know the secret behind exposure—habituation to the thing you fear—you're ready to use this powerful technique to conquer your anxiety. There are three key steps to using exposure. In the next sections, we'll walk you through these steps on your path toward a calmer pregnancy and postpartum experience:

1. Developing your exposure hierarchy.

2. Choosing the most effective method of exposure.

3. Practicing exposure until you are habituated to the experience.

One Step at a Time: Developing Your Exposure Hierarchy

The idea of eliminating familiar avoidance or safety behaviors, no matter how ineffective they are in the long run, may sound scary. But remember that you will be facing these fears gradually, starting with the things that bother you least. With practice on these initial tasks, soon you will be staring down your bigger fears with confidence and determination.

Start by considering your anxiety on a scale of 0 to 100. An anxiety level of 100 would mean the most distressing situation or thought you can imagine, while a 0 would indicate no anxiety at all. A level of 50 would represent a moderate level of anxiety or distress that is challenging but still relatively tolerable. When estimating your anxiety level, keep in mind that you are guessing at the discomfort you would feel if you were exposed to this situation, object, or thought without engaging in any avoidance or safety behaviors. Try to come up with items that create a range of anxiety levels, from low to high. Aim to put at least ten items on your exposure hierarchy, but don't worry if you have more or less.

As an example, Jan's exposure list is on the next page. Remember, Jan feared the impact of her actions on the health of her unborn baby, even though her doctor had approved her activities.

Jan's Exposure Hierarchy	
Situation/Thought	**Anxiety**
Taking acetaminophen or an antacid	100
Eating tuna once a week	85
Shaking hands with someone during flu season	80
Having lunch at the home of a friend who has two house cats	75
Standing near the microwave	70
Putting gas in the car	65
Drinking a cup of coffee	40
Walking near the paint section at a home improvement store	35

As another example, here is Maria's exposure hierarchy. Even though things were going fine in the present, Maria worried uncontrollably about her family's future.

Maria's Exposure Hierarchy	
Situation/Thought	**Anxiety**
My baby will have a birth defect.	100
I won't be able to handle labor and delivery.	90
What if I am not a good mother?	85
My husband could lose his job someday.	80
What if we get into a car accident?	70
I won't know how to take care of my baby.	65
What if our marriage can't take the strain of a baby?	55
I'll never be able to juggle home and work responsibilities.	55
What if our new toys have lead paint in them?	40

Now you give it a try. You may find it easiest to start with an anchor point: a situation or worry that you have been avoiding and would cause you a great deal of distress if you were to confront it. You can make that the top item on your hierarchy, with an anxiety level of 100. Next, think of something that would cause you only a moderate degree of anxiety to face and make that your midpoint, or 50. Now list your remaining feared situations or thoughts based on whether they would be easier or harder to confront than your anchor items.

Your Exposure Hierarchy	
Situation/Thought	**Anxiety**

Exposure Types: Finding a Strategy That Works for You

There are three different types of exposure that you may find helpful, depending on your particular anxiety symptoms.

Real-Life Exposure

A *real-life exposure* means entering into a situation that you find frightening, such as going to a crowded grocery store, visiting a friend who has a cat, driving a car, or using a knife to chop vegetables. Your own fears will determine what real-life exposures are appropriate for you.

Imaginal Exposure

When your fears are not easily addressed in real life or when actually approaching situations or objects would be too anxiety provoking at first, you can use *imaginal exposure* instead. As the name suggests, an imaginal exposure is one using your imagination. You might use this type of exposure for imagining bad things happening to yourself or a loved one, accidentally poisoning someone's food, or hitting someone with your car, for example. To do an imaginal exposure, you can write out, make an audio recording of, and repeatedly listen to a description of your feared scenario until your anxiety level comes down.

Physical Symptom Exposure

The third type of exposure, *physical symptom exposure,* is usually performed when someone is fearful of certain bodily sensations or symptoms, like those experienced during panic attacks. It involves intentionally creating feared but harmless symptoms like a racing heart or shortness of breath in order to become accustomed to these feelings; you might do things like walking fast, taking the stairs, or tensing muscles. If you are pregnant, this type of exposure will require clearance from your obstetrician before you engage in it.

> ### ~ COMMON QUESTION ~
> #### Won't exposure harm my baby?
>
> Some women worry that, if they don't avoid situations or thoughts that upset them, the anxiety that ensues will harm their health or that of their unborn baby. As we discussed in chapter 1, it is true that chronic stress and anxiety may lead to pregnancy problems, but this is different from the short-term rise in anxiety that we are discussing. In fact, you are probably at least as anxious in your constant battle to avoid and cope with these fears as you would be confronting them! And this chronic stress may have far more damaging effects on your and your baby's health. We propose that you instead apply the energy you've been using to avoid your fears to overcoming them. If you have concerns about using exposure therapy as a strategy for decreasing your anxiety, be sure to discuss them with your obstetrician.

Practice Exposure

Now that you've created your hierarchy and understand the different types of exposure, the next step is to practice. You can turn to part 3 of this book for more details on how exposure can be applied to your specific fears, or you can begin your practice now. Use the following guidelines to start facing your fears and conquering your anxiety:

1. Begin by selecting an item low on your hierarchy. It should be something challenging but not overwhelming. Usually something that is rated at about a 30 or 40 anxiety level is a good place to start, but you should begin at a point that feels right for you.

2. Decide whether your fear is best addressed by using real-life, imaginal, or physical symptom exposure. We've summarized the three types of exposures and their usefulness in the chart on the next page.

Type of Exposure	Common Uses
Real-life exposure	Directly confronting situations, thoughts, or images that make you anxious
Imaginal exposure	Confronting a fear that is not easily replicated in real life, or as a stepping-stone to real-life exposures
Physical symptom exposure	Confronting a bodily sensation, such as shortness of breath or racing heart, that triggers anxiety

3. Practice confronting your feared situation, thought, or sensation until your anxiety diminishes by at least half. So, if you start out with an exposure that you've rated as a 40 on your anxiety scale, try to focus on the exposure, without distracting yourself, until your anxiety decreases to about a 20. The anxiety level should come down during each exposure exercise. You will also notice that your anxiety may start out, or peak, a bit lower each time you practice.

4. Stay with the item until it causes you only mild or no anxiety, and then move up to the next item on your hierarchy and repeat the process. Everyone responds differently, so it may take you only a few days of practice with an item before you are ready to move on, or it may take a week or longer.

5. Continue to confront your fears until you have completed all items on your hierarchy.

Exercise: Practice Exposures

Use the steps above to begin confronting your feared situations. Don't worry if it is hard at first—you can do it! Stay with it and you'll see your anxiety begin to decrease over time. Remember to refrain from using any unhealthy coping strategies during your exposure practice—you want to get the most benefit from your efforts. If you have any concerns about the safety of confronting any items on your list, be sure to ask your obstetrician.

Why Do Exposure?

Our clients frequently ask us this important question. If you are bothered by something, what's wrong with just avoiding it or thinking about something else? It's a logical approach. But there are several reasons avoidance doesn't work, especially for anxiety. For one, what happens when you try to *not* think about something? You end up thinking about it even more, right? If I told you not to think about a pink elephant right now, chances are that a big, bright, rosy pachyderm would be the first thing to come to your mind. In fact, the more you try to not think about it, the more likely that elephant is to lumber through your mind.

But even if you could manage to do it, there are other pitfalls that come from trying to avoid thoughts or situations that worry or frighten you. It's human nature to want to avoid things that are unpleasant or that cause discomfort, but doing so may actually increase your fears in the long run. This is because, by avoiding thoughts that upset you, you treat them as a real threat or danger and as things that should be avoided at all costs. This undermines your confidence in your ability to tolerate these thoughts and to manage your anxiety, which in turn makes the thoughts even more powerful and frightening.

Avoiding thoughts or situations also keeps you from learning that you really could face them and nothing bad would happen. Along the same lines, the more you avoid certain worries or situations now, the more likely you are to avoid them in the future, setting up a vicious circle of anxiety and avoidance.

Tips for Successful Exposure

- Practice your exposure daily. Doing it sporadically won't work; it will only mean that you maintain the same high levels of anxiety. Make your efforts count!

- Be sure to stick with it. People are sometimes tempted to quit the exposure process early on, because experiencing anxiety can be unpleasant. Often they discontinue the exercise right when their anxiety has reached its peak, just before it's about to subside. It only *feels* like the anxiety will never end. Hang in there—it will go down with time.

- If you are using imaginal exposure, make your scenario as vivid and as specific as possible. Include details about the sounds, smells, sights, thoughts, and feelings involved. Write the scenario in the first person and in present tense, as if it were actually happening to you right now.

- Be sure to use your hierarchy to determine how to pace your exposures. Always pick something that is challenging but not overwhelming. When an exposure becomes easy, move up your hierarchy to the next one.

- When you eliminate an unhealthy coping behavior, make sure you don't substitute another one. This includes new behaviors that serve the same function as the one you eliminated.

- If you notice that your anxiety doesn't decrease, look closely for any subtle avoidance, distraction, or other behaviors that you may be engaging in. In the long run, they end up maintaining, not lessening, your anxiety.

- Review part 3 of this book for ways to apply exposures to your specific anxiety symptoms.

Next Steps

In this chapter, you've learned two key strategies for beating your anxiety—exposure and response prevention. By refraining from avoidance or unhealthy coping strategies and confronting the situations, thoughts, or physical sensations you fear, you can take major strides toward a calmer and more peaceful experience of motherhood. Continue practicing the techniques described in this chapter or turn to part 3 of this book for information on how to apply this strategy to specific anxiety problems, like panic attacks, obsessive-compulsive symptoms, worry, and post-traumatic stress.

Key Points

- Exposure—directly confronting your fears—is a key tool in overcoming your anxiety.

- Exposure works through habituation, your body's natural way of adjusting to anxiety.

- In exposure therapy, feared situations, thoughts, and sensations are confronted gradually and repeatedly for the best results.

- There are three types of exposure: real-life, imaginal, and physical symptom exposures.

- When you are engaging in exposure activities, remember that preventing any unhealthy coping behaviors, such as checking, repeating, or reassurance seeking, is critical to success.

- It is normal to feel apprehensive about the process of exposure but, when completed, it can be a very powerful and long-lasting antidote to anxiety.

CHAPTER 7

Learn to Solve Problems & Prioritize Your Time

The journey through pregnancy, childbirth, and parenting is an overwhelming prospect for anyone. You may wonder how some women seem to navigate this maternity maze effortlessly, efficiently creating a birth plan, choosing a pediatrician, and decorating the nursery, while others become paralyzed with anxiety. It may seem as if some women are just naturally born with the ability to juggle tasks and get things done; however, problem solving and time management are simply learned *skills*. No one is born knowing them but anyone can learn how, just like learning to ride a bike or spell your name! In this chapter, you'll learn an effective strategy to solve problems and key ways to manage your time more effectively; in the process, you will increase your self-confidence and lower your anxiety and stress.

Problem Solving Made Easy

The term *problem orientation* refers to how you think and feel about your problems as well as how you assess your problem-solving skills. Researchers have found that a negative problem orientation is associated with worry (Dugas and Ladouceur 2000) and with depression during pregnancy and the postpartum phase (Elliott et al. 1996). It seems that women with a negative problem orientation do have problem-solving skills but just have less confidence in their problem-solving abilities. So, though you might not ever be a multitasking Martha Stewart, the good news is that you can be a relaxed mom who has learned to prioritize and solve problems effectively. You can use these skills to address the many challenges of motherhood that lie before you.

Identify Productive Worries

Problems during pregnancy and the postpartum period come in many shapes and sizes, as you may know. Some are outlandish worries and fears of things we can't control. These types of anxiety are better addressed by other techniques described in this book, like cognitive restructuring or exposure therapy. The problem-solving approach we describe in this chapter works best when used with a *productive* worry or concern—a worry that is plausible, current, and solvable. This means that the concern is realistic and could actually happen, it is based in the present or in the near future, and it is something that you could control or solve if you tried.

Exercise: Identify Productive Worries

Knowing the difference between productive and unproductive worries is vital because it allows you to choose the correct strategy to address your anxiety. Problem solving only works with productive worries—those that are plausible, current, and solvable. Take a look at the following concerns and put a check mark next to the ones that are productive:

☐ What if I gain too much weight during pregnancy?

☐ My house is so cluttered that there's no room for the baby's crib.

☐ I need to find a good pediatrician.

☐ I might not know what to do during labor.

☐ What if my spouse dies in a car accident?

☐ I don't know whether to choose a daycare center or nanny.

☐ What if my baby has a rare birth defect?

How did you do? Were you able to identify which thoughts are current and plausible and which were future oriented and unrealistic? If you had trouble, consider these questions: Is this likely to happen? Are there any possible solutions to the problem? Is there anything that you could do about it today to make a change? How about within the next week? If the answer to these questions is no, then it is likely to be an unproductive or future-oriented worry. In the above exercise, concerns about birth defects and losing your spouse in a car accident are examples of worries that are unproductive, future oriented, and out of your control. The others can be addressed using the following problem-solving steps.

Problem-Solving Steps

1. **Define the problem and goal:** Define the key elements of the problem. Be as specific as possible. Be sure to also write what you would like to be different.

2. **Generate possible solutions:** Write down every possible solution you can imagine. Include any possible options, no matter how silly they may seem.

3. **Choose the best solution:** Pick the solution that you think has the best chance of success and seems most workable.

4. **Break down the solution:** Break down that solution into smaller steps that would be needed to achieve the goal.

Problem Solving in Action

One of our clients, Ella, was seven months pregnant and fearful that she would panic during delivery. Her problem-solving steps looked like this:

1. Define the problem and goal.
   Problem: I may not know what to expect or how to cope with the pain during labor and delivery.
   Goal: I would like to feel calm and knowledgeable while delivering my son.

2. Generate possible solutions.

   - Read a book on labor and delivery.

   - Take a childbirth class.

   - Ask my "mom" friends what to *really* expect.

   - Ignore this worry and hope that I will do fine.

   - Learn anxiety management or Lamaze techniques.

   - Hire a birth coach or doula.

   - Bring my labor and delivery book along so I can learn as I go.

3. Choose the best solution. Ella decided that many of these solutions were good ideas and might help, but she decided to start by taking a childbirth class. She chose this option because it was easy to accomplish and she felt she learned better from having things explained to her than from reading about them.

4. Break the solution down into manageable steps. Below are the steps Ella decided to take:

   a. Ella looked on the Internet and asked her obstetrician to recommend a childbirth class.

   b. She called to find out when the class was held.

   c. She picked a date that fit her schedule and registered for the class.

   d. She attended the class, learned what to expect, and practiced the strategies the instructor taught in order to deal with her anxiety.

Now it's your turn. Pick a concern that has been on your mind and write it in the space below:

_____

_____

_____

Before you go on, take a close look and make sure it is a productive worry or concern. Make a check mark next to the statements below that are true.

☐ Is it realistic or probable?

☐ Is it happening currently or in the near future?

☐ Can I do anything about it?

Did you check all three of the above statements? If so, great! Now take that problem and solve it by following the same steps that Ella used.

1. Define the problem and goal._____

   _____

   _____

   _____

2. Generate possible solutions.

   • _____

   • _____

   • _____

   • _____

   • _____

   • _____

3. Choose the best solution. _____

   _____

   _____

   ☐ Can I achieve this solution?

   ☐ Does it address my problem?

   ☐ Will it have a good chance of working?

4. Break the solution down into manageable steps.

a. _____

b. _____

c. _____

d. _____

e. _____

5. Now do it!

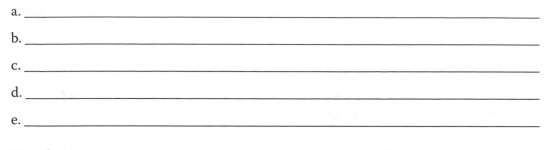

Exercise: Use Problem Solving in Your Everyday Life

Look for ways to apply problem solving in your everyday life. Begin by choosing productive worries and then simply use the steps above to solve them! You may find that this process is tedious or difficult at first. But with practice you'll be able to go through it efficiently and effectively. Over time, you'll develop more confidence in your ability to use your problem-solving skills and you'll find that you're able to eliminate many of the worries and tasks on your list.

Finding the Time

If you find that your newly polished problem-solving skills are working but you just have too many concerns or tasks to address, prioritizing the items on your list may help. We all sometimes feel as though there are just too many things to do and not nearly enough time to do them. This is especially true during pregnancy and the postpartum period. Can you think of times in the past month when you rushed to finish a project or a task? Were there times when you didn't do something important because you couldn't find the time? If you are pregnant or a new mom, we already know your answer to these questions!

You *can* learn to manage your time. And doing so will lessen your anxiety. Research has shown that building time-management skills decreases avoidance, procrastination, and worry (Van Eerde 2003). There is enough time to finish important tasks, meet goals, and do at least *most* of the things you want—if you prioritize and manage your time.

Effective Time Management

Below we'll describe an effective time management approach. This strategy consists of four steps:

1. Develop awareness.

2. Analyze how you spend your time.

3. Identify your priorities.

4. Plan your days.

Step One: Develop Awareness

Most people think that they have a handle on where their time goes, but many are unaware of time they waste on unnecessary or unproductive tasks. Before you can improve how you spend your time, you need to look at what you're doing with it now.

For the next week, closely monitor your activities using the Daily Activity Form below. Be sure to make extra copies so you have enough sheets for the whole week and also to use for exercises later in the chapter. Or, if you prefer, you can purchase a daily appointment calendar or use a notebook to create your own. Tracking your time will give you a detailed idea of where you spend your time and whether adjustments might help. Be sure to keep track of how much time you spend sleeping, eating, commuting, watching television, and running errands. Include as much detail as possible. Keep your notebook or calendar with you and record activities as soon as you complete them. Don't rely on your memory or wait until the end of the day to fill out the form. In order for this exercise to be useful, you need to create an accurate picture of your schedule.

You might believe you don't need to do this, because you already know where your time goes. As an experiment, write down the amount of time you think you'll spend doing things like sleeping, eating, watching TV, running errands, making phone calls, and using the Internet during the next week. Then, monitor your time for at least a few days and see how close your guesses were. Our clients usually find they weren't very accurate in their estimates. In fact, they're often shocked at the amount of time they spend on things like watching TV or using the Internet.

> **⋅• COMMON QUESTION ~**
> **What if I'm too busy to do this?**
>
> If you're like our clients, keeping such close track of your schedule probably sounds overwhelming to you. Keep in mind that this task is only temporary. You don't have to do this exercise for the rest of your life—you just have to do it for one week. And by spending the time now, you'll gain more time in the future. Consider it an investment in decreasing your worry, anxiety, and stress; it is the first step to gaining more control over how you use your time.

Daily Activity Form	
Time	**Activity**
6:00 a.m.	
6:30 a.m.	
7:00 a.m.	
7:30 a.m.	
8:00 a.m.	
8:30 a.m.	
9:00 a.m.	
9:30 a.m.	
10:00 a.m.	
10:30 a.m.	
11:00 a.m.	
11:30 a.m.	
12:00 p.m.	
12:30 p.m.	
1:00 p.m.	
1:30 p.m.	
2:00 p.m.	
2:30 p.m.	
3:00 p.m.	
3:30 p.m.	
4:00 p.m.	
4:30 p.m.	
5:00 p.m.	
5:30 p.m.	
6:00 p.m.	
6:30 p.m.	
7:00 p.m.	
7:30 p.m.	

8:00 p.m.	
8:30 p.m.	
9:00 p.m.	
9:30 p.m.	
10:00 p.m.	
10:30 p.m.	
11:00 p.m.	
11:30 p.m.	
12:00 a.m.	
12:30 a.m.	
1:00 a.m.	
1:30 a.m.	
2:00 a.m.	
2:30 a.m.	
3:00 a.m.	
3:30 a.m.	
4:00 a.m.	
4:30 a.m.	
5:00 a.m.	
5:30 a.m.	

Step Two: Analyze How You Spend Your Time

Did you record your activities for the week? If not, do so before you move on. It's an essential step in managing your time better. By recording your activities, you can look at where your time went. Once you've recorded your activities, analyze how you spent your time, using the following steps:

1. Look at the activities you recorded over the past week. Can you group them into categories using the form below? Some possible categories include sleeping, eating, caring for your children, working, reading, watching TV, running errands, making phone calls, using the Internet, personal grooming or hygiene, cooking meals, doing household chores, commuting, and recreation. Use these categories as a start, but add other activities to the list if necessary.

Categories	Time Spent
Sleeping	
Eating	
Childcare	
Working	
Household chores	
Running errands	
Making phone calls	
Using the Internet	
Grooming	
Cooking meals	
Commuting	
Recreation	
Other:	
Total Time Spent	**168 hours**

2. Now, on the right side of that page, tally up how much time you spent over the past week doing activities in each category. Be sure that you account for all 168 hours in a week.

3. Were you surprised by your results? Did you spend more time on certain things than you thought you would? Was there anything you wish you'd done more of? How about less of? Did you spend any time doing unnecessary tasks? Was there anything that you wanted to get done but didn't? Record your answers here:

Wish I'd done more: Wish I'd done less:

_____   _____

_____   _____

_____   _____

_____   _____

Andrea was a client who used this step to reduce her anxiety and worry. As a new mom and a business executive with a hectic schedule, she found that she had trouble getting things done. As she went through her day, she frequently felt anxious and overwhelmed by the sheer number of tasks facing her. In an effort to improve her time management skills, Andrea monitored her activities for one week. When she tallied up the amount of time she spent on each type of activity, she discovered that many tasks, like searching the Internet, took much longer than she meant them to or were unnecessary altogether. This gave her hope that she could manage her time more effectively. By following the next two steps, she reevaluated her priorities and recaptured lost time. As a result, she was able to spend more time on things that were important to her, like reading to her new baby. These new skills helped Andrea dramatically reduce her anxiety and recapture time for things that she valued.

Step Three: Identify Your Priorities

Take a look at how you answered the questions in step two and consider those answers when planning your upcoming week. If, like many new moms, you found that you spent a lot of time in activities that were unnecessary while other important tasks went undone, you might find the following strategy helpful.

First, make a master list of things you want to accomplish. Don't spend too much time on this step, and don't worry if it isn't perfect—you can always add to this list as new goals or obligations arise. Now, think about each task on your list and decide whether it falls into one of the following categories:

High priority: extremely important and critical to complete today

Medium priority: very important, but not urgent that it be done today

Low priority: important and needs to be done, but not right away

If any tasks don't fit into one of these three categories—in other words, if they are unimportant or unnecessary—consider crossing them off your list altogether. In fact, you might even consider deleting the low-priority items from your list!

Brianna was a new, stay-at-home mom with a four-month-old baby girl, Caitlyn. Her list looked something like this:

Weekly Master Task List	Priority Category (High, Medium, Low)
Laundry	Medium
Exercise	High
Find music class for Caitlyn	Medium
Return phone calls	Medium
Change cable service	Low
Schedule oil change	Medium
Sort and organize baby clothes	Low

Buy diapers	High
Mail phone bill payment	High
Write thank-you notes	Medium
~~Choose and print pictures for notes~~	~~Medium~~

Notice that Brianna only marked a few items on her list as "high priority" (buying diapers, mailing the phone bill payment, and exercising). She chose these items because they had strict deadlines, were necessary, or were of high value and importance to her. You'll notice that she crossed off her list the task of printing photographs to include in her thank-you notes. Though she felt this would be a nice touch, she decided to delete it because she had already sent out birth announcements with a photo and because it was keeping her from completing the more-important task of writing and sending the thank-you notes. She found that freeing herself from this task allowed her to complete the important tasks and decreased her feelings of stress and anxiety.

Now go ahead and fill out your own weekly master task list.

Weekly Master Task List	Priority Category (High, Medium, Low)

Step Four: Plan Your Days

Now, using your planner or copies of the blank Daily Activity Form, write any scheduled appointments, meetings, or other activities for the week that have a firm beginning and ending time. If any of these require travel, be sure to block off time for that too. Next, take high-priority items from your Weekly Master Task List and put them into the free slots in your schedule. You don't want to have too many high-priority items—if it seems you have a lot in one day, say more than two or three, consider whether you are exaggerating their importance and urgency. If any free time remains, take medium-priority tasks from the list and schedule them. Consider crossing low-priority tasks off your list, and only add them to the schedule if time remains after you've accounted for high- and medium-priority tasks.

> ### ~ COMMON QUESTION ~
> **What if my baby doesn't want to cooperate with this schedule?**
>
> If you are a new mom, or if you are pregnant but have small children at home, you may need to be more flexible. Instead of scheduling specific times for high-priority items, just write them at the top of your schedule for that day and fit them in whenever you can. Keep in mind that during the first few months of motherhood your high-priority items may be things like napping, showering, or eating lunch. Be realistic. Expecting too much from yourself during this time won't make you more productive; instead, it will only interfere with your ability to get things done and make you more stressed and anxious.

Scheduling and Time-Saving Tips for New Moms

No other time in your life will be quite so wonderful and chaotic all at once. Remember to cut yourself some slack and use the following tips to maximize your time:

- Be flexible. If you are accustomed to being organized, the chaos that now surrounds you may be difficult to take. Remember, it is only temporary. Things will improve with time. Try to go with the flow for now.

- Remember to be realistic about what you can accomplish, especially in those first few months after your baby arrives. If you can just manage to get a shower, you're doing great!

- Be careful in your estimates of how long activities will take you. When in doubt, allow for extra time.

- Delegate whenever you can. Don't be afraid to ask others for help. Be specific in your requests.

- Remember your priorities. It's okay to let some things go temporarily or take shortcuts in order to get the essential tasks done—so give yourself permission to order carry-out food, use paper plates, and have groceries delivered.

- Don't be afraid to say no. Turn down requests if you need to and take care of yourself and your baby first. Your friends and family will understand.

- Take your baby with you. Wear your baby in a sling or carrier while doing household tasks, or put her in a stroller so you can do errands together. Your baby will get to see new things and you will get things done.

- Designate "daddy time." Allow your partner some time each day to bond with your baby and give you a break.

- Leave time between tasks so you don't rush from one thing to another. Whenever possible, finish one activity before moving on to the next. Scheduling fewer tasks but making sure to finish each one will leave you feeling more relaxed and may actually improve your productivity in the long run.

- Allow for travel time and plan for the worst-case scenario. Include time for congested traffic, stormy weather, and last-minute diaper changes.

- Don't forget to schedule time for yourself! In the long run, you'll be more productive if you allow some time of your own. Consider swapping babysitting duties with another mom, asking a friend or family member to step in, or hiring a sitter.

As a pregnant or new mom, you are assigned the very important job of nurturing your baby's development. If some other things get put on the back burner, so be it. Chores and errands can often wait, but your baby will only be little once. Enjoy your time together and be sure to take care of yourself. The rest will fall into place.

Next Steps

Continue practicing these skills. Effective problem solving and time management will come in handy on your journey to motherhood and beyond. Keep in mind, though, that these strategies are just one piece of the puzzle. Use them, along with the other skills you've learned in this book, as you move on to part 3; there, you will find instructions for addressing specific anxiety problems you may experience like panic, worry, obsessions, and post-traumatic stress.

Key Points

- Learning problem-solving and time-management skills can decrease your anxiety and help you address the many new tasks that go along with pregnancy and motherhood.

- Productive worries can be addressed using problem-solving strategies.

- Analyzing the way you spend your time and identifying your priorities can help you to manage your time better and get more done.

- During pregnancy and the postpartum period, you may need to lower productivity expectations and simply focus on caring for yourself and your baby.

PART 3

Applying Cognitive
Behavioral Therapy to Specific
Anxiety Problems

CHAPTER 8

Manage Panic Attacks & Other Physical Symptoms

Pregnancy is a time of excitement, anticipation, and change. With the arrival of your little one, your world transforms in ways you never imagined. But, along with the amazing experiences of pregnancy and new motherhood, the emotional and physical changes you may go through can be taxing or even downright overwhelming at times. Heart palpitations, shortness of breath, nausea, dizziness, and frequent urination—all these symptoms can be part of a normal pregnancy. Unfortunately, because these symptoms can be uncomfortable and sometimes frightening, in some women they can trigger anxiety and panic attacks or can worsen an existing panic disorder.

In this chapter, you'll learn how to identify symptoms of panic, manage your responses to physical changes, and rein in catastrophic misinterpretations of these sensations. Your step-by-step plan for dealing with panic attacks will guide you to recognize, accept, and cope with these symptoms and return your focus to the exciting time ahead of you. At the end of this chapter you'll also find helpful tips for dealing with common physical complaints that can cause anxiety during pregnancy.

What Is a Panic Attack?

A panic attack is a sudden, intense rush of fear that usually lasts about ten to fifteen minutes. As we mentioned in chapter 3, panic attacks can include frightening symptoms (American Psychiatric Association 2000), such as the following:

- Racing heart
- Lightheadedness or dizziness
- Numbness or tingling sensations
- Sweating

- Trembling

- Feeling short of breath

- Feeling of choking

- Chest pain or discomfort

- Nausea

- Fear of losing control or going crazy

- Fear of dying

- Chills or hot flashes

Panic attacks are common—about a third of the population report having experienced one or more panic attacks in their life (Norton, Dorward, and Cox 1986). Panic attacks can be triggered by a variety of stressful situations or they can occur out of the blue. Some people who have panic attacks go on to develop *panic disorder*, a condition in which the attacks appear to occur spontaneously; these attacks provoke fear, worry, or avoidance of situations that might trigger another panic attack. Panic disorder happens more frequently in women, with about 5 percent of women meeting criteria for panic disorder at some point in their lifetime (Kessler et al. 1994). That's nearly 8 million women in the United States alone!

Panic in Pregnancy and the Postpartum Phase

It's not entirely clear how pregnancy impacts panic. Some researchers have suggested that a preexisting tendency to have panic attacks can actually lessen during pregnancy, possibly due to the calming effects of progesterone, particularly in women with mild anxiety symptoms (Cohen et al. 1994). For other women, the frequency of their panic attacks may remain unchanged.

For still others, symptoms can worsen or develop during this time (Hertzberg and Wahlbeck 1999), perhaps because the physical changes that occur during pregnancy may lower the threshold for experiencing panic. For instance, as your pregnancy progresses you may experience mild breathlessness because your growing baby compresses your diaphragm. As your uterus expands and pushes up against your diaphragm, it crowds your lungs and limits the amount of air you can take in. Simultaneously, your respiratory system is adapting in order to carry large amounts of oxygen to the placenta, and hormone changes are causing you to breathe more frequently. As a result, you may take in more oxygen than you are using, leading to a subtle but chronic hyperventilation that can cause you to feel short of breath. These changes are not dangerous, but they can feel scary. Misinterpretation

~ COMMON QUESTION ~

What if my breathlessness is severe?

Mild breathlessness is common in pregnancy. However, you should discuss any severe shortness of breath with your obstetrician, because it may indicate a more serious problem. Your doctor will likely rule out things like thyroid dysfunction, anemia, and preeclampsia before diagnosing you with panic (Ross and McLean 2006).

of these new breathing patterns and sensations can result in anxiety, which can then escalate to panic.

It is also common to see anxiety strike in the postpartum period, either for the first time or as a worsening of existing panic symptoms. In fact, many women have reported that their panic emerged during the first twelve weeks after birth (Sholomskas et al. 1993) or that their panic symptoms got worse when they weaned their babies (Northcott and Stein 1994).

What does this mean for you? If you have a history of panic attacks, you may be particularly vulnerable to a recurrence or escalation of your symptoms during the postpartum period. Even if you've never had panic attacks before, the physical, emotional, and situational changes of pregnancy and new motherhood may lead to panic attacks. In either case, the strategies outlined in this chapter will be helpful to you.

How to Tell if Your Symptoms Are Related to Pregnancy

There is quite a bit of overlap between the physical changes of pregnancy and anxiety symptoms. As you can see from the pregnancy-related thoughts and feelings listed below, these symptoms can be easily mistaken for anxiety (Kelly and Little 2001).

Normal Pregnancy Changes

- Increased heart rate, occasional palpitations
- Awareness of breathing or shortness of breath
- Increased salivation
- Heartburn
- Nausea and vomiting
- Dizziness when changing position
- Sweating
- Numbness associated with muscle strain or swelling
- Hot or cold flashes
- Concerns about health or care of child
- Nesting behavior, avoidance of activities or situations that could harm the baby
- Increased frequency of urination

However, if you find yourself becoming anxious about many different things, if your physical sensations are extreme, or if your fears are overwhelming, you may be experiencing anxiety or panic. Use the checklist on the following page to determine whether your symptoms are the result of normal pregnancy changes or a sign of anxiety or panic.

Tracking Your Panic Symptoms

The first crucial step in beating panic is to know your symptoms. You might already feel as though you are intimately familiar with these uncomfortable physical sensations and the scary thoughts that accompany them, but you may be surprised at what you find when you look closely. In order to apply the strategies in this chapter fully, you will want to have a clear idea of the pattern of your symptoms and the situations that trigger them. Place a check mark next to the panic symptoms that you usually experience:

☐ Racing heart　　　　　　　　　　☐ Chest pain or discomfort

☐ Lightheadedness or dizziness　　　☐ Nausea

☐ Numbness or tingling sensations　☐ Fear of losing control

☐ Sweating　　　　　　　　　　　　☐ Fear of going crazy

☐ Trembling　　　　　　　　　　　☐ Fear of dying

☐ Feeling short of breath　　　　　☐ Feelings of unreality

☐ Feeling of choking　　　　　　　☐ Chills or hot flashes

Understand Your Panic Components

Before you go on, let's be sure you understand the different components of anxiety and panic, and the variables that are important for you to track. Anxiety and panic consist of three main factors: the physical, the cognitive, and the behavioral.

The Physical Component

The physical symptoms of panic are hard to miss. As we showed in the exercise above, they include things like shortness of breath, racing heart, numbness or tingling, sweating, dizziness, nausea, and chest pain. You are already well aware of this component if you are experiencing panic.

The Cognitive Component

The cognitive, or thinking, piece of panic may be a little less obvious to you, particularly because people tend to focus more on the intense physical discomfort associated with it. However, the cognitive component of panic plays a critical role in the escalation of anxiety. Common thoughts that run through your mind during intense anxiety or panic attacks may relate to losing control, going crazy, or even dying.

The Behavioral Component

The behavioral part of panic is what you do when you are anxious or panicky, or what you may do to try to avoid these feelings. Frequently, people will avoid situations where it's difficult to escape or modify their behavior to make it easier to escape if panic strikes. For example, you may avoid going to stores during peak times when lines may be long or you may sit near an exit at the movies. Avoidance can also be mental, like distracting yourself from your nervousness by listening to the radio or carrying on a conversation. It can also take the form of "safety" behaviors like carrying medications, water, or a cell phone with you at all times.

Sylvie, who was six months pregnant with her first child, examined her panic symptoms and broke down the components as follows:

Physical	Cognitive	Behavioral
Heart races	What is happening?	Avoid climbing stairs when home alone
Stomach churns	Something is wrong with the baby.	Lie down
Hands shake	I could pass out.	Keep phone next to me at all times
Feel like I can't breathe	I might be dying.	Call my husband to come home
Hot flashes		

Now, think about one of your own recent episodes of panic. Consider what physical symptoms you had during these times, what thoughts ran through your mind, and what you did to make yourself feel better or to avoid future panic attacks. Record your anxiety and panic components in the appropriate columns below:

Physical	Cognitive	Behavioral

How Your Anxiety Components Interact

Although it may seem as if panic attacks happen suddenly and out of the blue, your anxiety components actually work together and build on one another to produce panic-level anxiety. A panic attack may start with subtle physical sensations that then get worse as you react with anxious thoughts or behavior. For instance, when Sylvie looked closely she found that her panic attacks usually started with a feeling of mild breathlessness (physical) when walking, climbing stairs, or performing household chores. This breathlessness would trigger the thought "What is happening to me? I might pass out" (cognitive). Sylvie then felt even more anxious and her heart would begin to race and her hands would tremble (physical). This led her to call her husband to come home from work (behavioral). While she waited for him to arrive, she would lie down and scan her body for any further sensations (behavioral). She would notice that she felt a little nauseated, and as she focused on her nausea (physical) she would worry, "What if something is wrong with the baby?" (cognitive). She would then begin to feel dizzy and warm (physical), clutching the telephone in case of emergency (behavioral), convinced that something was terribly wrong (cognitive). You can see that what started out as a mild nuisance common to normal pregnancy (shortness of breath) quickly escalated to a panic attack with the contribution of catastrophic thoughts and avoidance or safety behaviors.

Exercise: Track Your Panic

For the next week, keep track of your panic attacks using the form on the next page. Photocopy as many as you need to record the date, time and situation in which each of your panic attacks occur. Write down any triggers that you notice and circle the intensity level of your anxiety. Check off any physical sensations that you experience and write down any anxious thoughts or behaviors.

Looking back at your records over the past week, ask yourself these questions:

Did you notice any thoughts that triggered your anxiety? _____

_____

Was panic more likely to occur in certain situations? _____

_____

Was any physical sensation or thought most likely to initiate your panic attacks? _____

_____

What were you afraid might happen? _____

_____

How did you react? _____

_____

Did you do something to try to escape? _____

_____

Did you avoid a situation because you thought it might trigger a panic attack? _____

_____

Panic Attack Record

Date and Time: _____

Situation or Trigger: _____

Anxiety Level
(circle)

0	10	20	30	40	50	60	70	80	90	100

Not Anxious   **Moderately Anxious**   **Very Anxious**

☐ Racing heart   ☐ Chest pain or discomfort

☐ Lightheadedness or dizziness   ☐ Nausea

☐ Numbness or tingling sensations   ☐ Fear of losing control

☐ Sweating   ☐ Fear of going crazy

☐ Trembling   ☐ Fear of dying

☐ Feeling short of breath   ☐ Chills or hot flashes

☐ Feeling of choking

What I thought: _____

_____

_____

_____

What I did: _____

_____

_____

_____

Your Five-Step Plan to Managing Panic

Now that you understand more about anxiety and how your symptoms interact to produce panic attacks, you're ready to use the skills you learned in part 2 of this book to reverse the panic cycle. In this section, we'll describe five key steps to lessening panic during pregnancy or the postpartum phase:

1. Educate yourself.

2. Use relaxation skills.

3. Challenge your anxious thoughts.

4. Confront your feared situations.

5. Confront feared physical sensations.

Step One: Educate Yourself

We've mentioned some of the physical changes that commonly overlap with anxiety, but it is important for you to understand exactly what is normal to expect from your body during pregnancy and the postpartum period. Women who have panic attacks have a tendency to be highly vigilant about physical changes in their bodies and to misinterpret these symptoms as dangerous or harmful. Because at no other time in your life will you undergo so many physical changes, they can leave you vulnerable to developing panic attacks.

If you haven't done so already, find a trusted reference guide that you can turn to when you have questions about the physical sensations you are experiencing. Try to use just one comprehensive text for this purpose; using multiple resources can lead to confusion, over analysis and increased anxiety. See appendix B for suggested sources of information. If you choose to use the Internet for this purpose, choose one reputable, professional site rather than searching Internet forums and blogs for answers. Remember, anyone can post information on the Internet and you cannot always be certain of what is opinion rather than fact. When in doubt, contact your obstetrician's office. Don't be afraid to call with questions; most practices will be happy to address any worries you may have.

When you really understand what to expect from pregnancy and in the postpartum period, you will be less likely to fear your physical sensations and it will be easier for you to challenge any anxious thoughts you have about them.

Step Two: Use Relaxation Skills

The second step in beating panic attacks is to work on your relaxation skills. In chapter 4, you learned that relaxation is a skill that you can work to master. Though you can use any of the techniques described in chapter 4, we find that our clients who suffer panic attacks benefit most from using diaphragmatic breathing to counter the effects of anxiety. Once you've practiced this skill and feel comfortable using it, you can use it any time you notice anxiety starting to build.

Exercise: Practice Diaphragmatic Breathing

Look back to chapter 4 and review the instructions for diaphragmatic breathing. Continue to practice this technique each day until you are comfortable with it. At that point, you will be ready to use this skill in situations where you find yourself becoming anxious.

Tips for Dealing with Shortness of Breath During Pregnancy

The breathlessness that can occur during normal pregnancy can often be misinterpreted as harmful and cause your anxiety to escalate, leading to panic attacks. If you find that shortness of breath is a trigger for your panic, use diaphragmatic breathing skills and also try the following suggestions:

- **Maintain good posture.** Standing or sitting up straight, with your shoulders back and down, will help you to breathe better. Remember that during pregnancy your diaphragm is being crowded by your uterus, making it difficult for you to breathe. The more room you can give yourself to breathe by sitting and standing tall, the less breathless you will feel.

- **Practice yoga.** The gentle stretching of yoga can help you to prepare and to strengthen your body for labor and delivery. With its focus on steady and mindful breathing, yoga can also help you to be aware of your breath and improve your breathing technique.

- **Exercise.** Light aerobic exercise may improve your breathing and lead to less shortness of breath. Talk with your obstetrician about whether an exercise program would be right for you.

Step Three: Challenge Your Anxious Thoughts

In chapter 5, you learned about how your thoughts can influence your emotions. This is definitely the case with panic attacks. Hypervigilance about physical changes and misinterpretation of these cues is a key factor in the development of panic attacks. Though anxious thinking can involve many of the distortions listed in chapter 5, the main culprits that trigger panic attacks can generally be whittled down to two:

- **Overestimating probabilities.** This is just what it sounds like—overestimating the likelihood that something will happen. In the case of panic, you may be thinking that something bad is more likely to happen than it really is. For instance, when Christine was eight months pregnant she would experience intense anxiety when she became short of breath. She would immediately think, "I'm having a heart attack. I'm going to lose the baby."

- **Catastrophizing.** This distortion makes situations seem worse than they really are. Christine would engage in this type of thinking as well when thinking about her panic attacks and their perceived consequences. "If I have a panic attack, I won't be able to cope, so I need to have someone with me at all times. It would be terrible if I panicked in public. I'd be mortified."

Look closely at the thoughts you have written down on your Panic Attack Records. Do you notice any times when you might have been overestimating the probability of a bad outcome or exaggerating the negative consequences of a panic attack?

Changing Your Panic Thoughts

Now it's time to challenge those misinterpretations and lower your anxiety. In chapter 5, we described several techniques for changing your thinking. You can use any of those techniques that you like, but we have found that two techniques—examining the evidence, and countering catastrophic thinking—tend to work best in challenging overestimated probabilities and catastrophic thoughts.

Examine the Evidence

During a panic attack, we tend to treat our anxious thoughts as truths rather than as hypotheses that can be tested. The physical symptoms may be so intense that you think, "I am definitely having a heart attack this time," even though you have been fine all the other times you have experienced the same symptoms. Examining the evidence just means taking a look at all of the available information in order to "test out" whether your anxious thought is true. Rather than accept the scary thought as fact, ask yourself the following questions to see how realistic it really is:

- "What am I predicting will happen? Do I know for sure that it will come true?"

- "What evidence do I have for this prediction? "

- "Have I made similar predictions in the past? How often have they come true?"

- "Are there any other reasons I could be feeling this way?"

- "What is the evidence against this prediction?"

- "Which side is more convincing?"

- "What should I do now?"

Christine used this technique to challenge her fears that she was going to have a heart attack or lose her baby when she felt anxious. Her examination of the evidence looked like this:

Examining the Evidence
Anxious Thought: I am having a heart attack and will lose the baby.

- What am I predicting will happen? That I'll have a heart attack and lose my baby
  - Do I know for sure that it will come true? No.
- What evidence do I have for this prediction? I'm feeling short of breath and my heart is pounding.
- Have I made similar predictions in the past? Yes, I feel this way several times a week.
  - How often have they come true? I've never had a heart attack, and I'm still pregnant.
- Are there any other reasons I could be feeling this way? I guess my body is working pretty hard at being pregnant. Maybe I was walking too fast and that made me short of breath
- So, what is the evidence against this prediction?
  - I've felt this way many times before and never lost the baby.
  - I see my doctor often and she always examines me and tells me I am healthy.
  - The books I read tell me that shortness of breath is common in pregnancy, especially in the third trimester.
  - I don't have any symptoms of heart disease.
- Which side is more convincing? The evidence against.
- What should I do now? I could practice using my breathing techniques to lower my anxiety.

Now you try it! Look back at your Panic Attack Records and find a thought where you predicted a negative outcome. Use the form on the next page to ask yourself the questions Christine used to challenge her anxious thoughts.

Examining the Evidence

Anxious Thought: _____

- What am I predicting will happen? _____

    - Do I know for sure that it will come true? _____

- What evidence do I have for this prediction? _____

_____

- Have I made similar predictions in the past? _____

    - How often have they come true? _____

- Are there any other reasons I could be feeling this way? _____

_____

- So, what is the evidence against this prediction?

_____

_____

_____

- Which side is more convincing? _____

- What should I do now? _____

_____

Counter Catastrophic Thinking

To beat catastrophic thinking, you'll need to ask yourself questions that help you to evaluate your concerns in a realistic way. This strategy works best to address thoughts about how terrible it would be if a negative outcome occurred. Christine asked herself the following questions to combat her catastrophic thoughts:

- What is the worst thing that could happen?

- How likely is the worst-case scenario?

- What could I do to cope if the worst-case scenario did occur? How have I coped in the past?

- Would it really be as bad as I'm imagining?

- What are at least three other possible outcomes?

- How bad has it been in the past when I've had a panic attack?

She used the form below to test out her thought that it would be terrible to have a panic attack in public. As you can see, when she carefully considered the realistic consequences of panicking she realized that she had been exaggerating how awful the situation was.

Countering Catastrophic Thinking
Anxious Thought: It would be terrible if I panicked in public. I'd be mortified.

- What is the worst-case scenario? I would have a panic attack in front of others and they would notice that something was wrong.

- How likely is the worst-case scenario? It is possible. In the past, others have asked me if I'm okay.

- What could I do to cope if the worst-case scenario did occur? How have I coped in the past? I could find a quiet place do my diaphragmatic breathing exercises. In the past, all my panic attacks have passed within a few minutes.

- Would it really be as bad as I'm imagining? Maybe not. Usually people don't even notice that I'm anxious and, when they do, they are usually supportive.

- What are at least three other possible outcomes?

  - I have a panic attack and no one even notices.

  - I accept that sometimes others might see me being anxious.

  - I find a quiet spot to breathe until my panic passes.

- How bad has it been in the past when I've had a panic attack? It is pretty uncomfortable and I don't like it, but nothing terrible has happened.

- What is the most likely outcome? I may sometimes have panic attacks in public but I can cope with it, and, if anyone even notices, I can just deal with my temporary feelings of embarrassment.

Now take one of your thoughts from your Panic Attack Records that you think may have involved catastrophic thinking and use the form below to test it out.

Countering Catastrophic Thinking

Anxious Thought: _____

- What is the worst-case scenario? _____

  _____

- How likely is the worst-case scenario? _____

- What could I do to cope if the worst-case scenario did occur? _____

  _____

- How have I coped in the past? _____

  _____

- Would it really be as bad as I'm imagining? _____

  _____

- What are at least three other possible outcomes?

  - _____

  - _____

  - _____

- How bad has it been in the past when I've had a panic attack? _____

  _____

- What is the most likely outcome? _____

  _____

Exercise: Challenge Your Panic Thoughts

After you have practiced countering some of your previous thoughts, you will be ready to use this strategy when you are anxious. Examine the evidence or counter catastrophic thinking whenever you find yourself feeling panicky. Don't worry if it is hard at first. Keep at it and it will get easier. Eventually you will be able to challenge those thoughts without even writing them down!

Step Four: Confront Feared Situations

In chapter 6, we discussed exposure therapy and how helpful it can be for dealing with anxiety problems such as panic. In this step, you will learn how to apply real-life exposures to confront any situations that you have been avoiding.

Using Real-Life Exposure to Beat Panic Attacks

One of the main reasons for using exposure is to teach yourself that your fearful predictions just aren't accurate. Though you may be using the methods in step three quite effectively to counter your anxious thoughts, you may have some lingering doubts. Directly confronting the situations that you fear is the only way for you to believe, without a shadow of a doubt, that your dire predictions won't come true. Avoiding situations where you may feel panicky only prevents you from learning that these situations are actually safe and, worse, it undermines your confidence that you can manage your anxiety.

Your Exposure Hierarchy

Look back at your exposure hierarchy in chapter 6. It should include any situations or places that you avoid or where you fear you'll panic. This could mean places that are difficult to escape from, like long lines, crowded stores, or theaters, or situations like driving, being away from home, or being alone. Remember to list your items in order of how much anxiety you would feel if you confronted them, with 100 being the worst possible anxiety, 0 being no anxiety, and 50 indicating moderate anxiety.

Christine's hierarchy looked like this:

Feared Situations	Anxiety
Driving alone over the Golden Gate Bridge in heavy traffic	100
Being in a crowded restaurant with a work colleague	90
Driving alone on a city street on a weekend	85
Driving with my husband in heavy traffic	85
Being in crowded mall alone, far from the entrance	75
Standing in line at a crowded grocery store alone	70
Shopping with my husband	60
Walking near my home alone without my cell phone	55
Walking near my home alone with my cell phone	40

Now that you've completed your hierarchy, select an item that's low on the list—something challenging but not overwhelming. Practice exposing yourself to that situation. With each situation, start by rating your actual anxiety on a scale of 0 to 100. Try to stay in the situation until your anxiety diminishes by about half. Leaving before you habituate will sabotage all the effort you are putting into facing your fears. Practice putting yourself in that situation as often as you can until it causes you only mild or no anxiety. Then move up to the next item on your hierarchy and repeat the process. For example, when Christine began by walking near her home with a cell phone, an exposure that she rated as a 40 on her anxiety scale, she kept walking that day until her anxiety decreased to about a 20. She repeated that exercise each day for about a week, by which time the activity no longer caused her much anxiety. She then moved on to walking *without* her cell phone and practiced that until she felt comfortable. She continued this way until she had addressed all the items on her list.

Christine found that as she approached some of the items on her hierarchy she was able to more clearly identify and tackle some of her anxious thoughts too. When she noticed that her thoughts were causing her anxiety to escalate or were interfering with her ability to follow through on the exposure, she went back to step three and used cognitive techniques to challenge those thoughts. For instance, when Christine set out to practice walking without her cell phone, she had the thought, "What if I don't bring the cell phone and something happens to the baby?" She felt anxious and guilty at first, but by examining the evidence for this probability overestimation she was able to lower her anxiety, recognize that the risk was small, and move on to the next item on her exposure hierarchy.

Step Five: Confront Feared Sensations

Now that you've confronted the situations you fear, you're ready to turn your attention to your physical sensations. With panic attacks, the fear of the bodily sensations you experience is a powerful element in perpetuating your anxiety. As we noted previously, women who panic tend to be hypervigilant to physical sensations or changes in their body. This means that you are literally searching your body for signs that something might be wrong. Because these possible signs can almost always be found if you look for them, especially during pregnancy, this leads to heightened anxiety and fear. This association between physical sensations and fear is strengthened by misinterpreting the significance of these symptoms, and soon you are on high alert for any signs of panic—noticing even the most subtle physical symptoms.

Physical Symptom Exposure

Earlier in this chapter, you identified the physical symptoms you often experience when you are panicky. Now it is time to reclaim your body and face these feared sensations head-on. Remember, physical symptom exposure involves intentionally creating feared but harmless sensations like a racing heart or shortness of breath so that you can become accustomed to these feelings. This exercise may include activities like walking fast, taking the stairs, or tensing muscles. As is the case with exposure to frightening situations, repeated practice in confronting feared sensations will result in lower anxiety, less fear, and fewer panic attacks.

Note: If you are pregnant, recovering from childbirth, or have any medical conditions, get clearance from your obstetrician before trying this type of exposure. He or she can guide you toward exercises you can safely do.

Your Hierarchy of Feared Sensations

When creating your hierarchy of physical symptom exposures, you start by identifying which sensations bother you the most and are most similar to your anxiety feelings. There are a number of exercises that you can perform to identify the ones that most closely mimic those that you fear during a panic attack. The idea is to engage in each of the exercises as fully as possibly to bring on the feared sensations.

Try each of the following exercises and record the results using the form below. In the first column, record which physical symptoms you noticed during the exercise. In the second column, rate your level of anxiety during the exercise from 0 (none) to 100 (high). In the third column, rate how similar your physical sensations during this exercise are to the physical symptoms you normally experience during a panic attack, from 0 (not similar) to 100 (very similar).

Sensation Induction Exercises

- Shake your head from side to side for thirty seconds (dizziness).

- Hold your breath for as long as you can, or for about thirty seconds (breathlessness, chest tightness).

- Spin in a chair for about one minute (dizziness, nausea).

- Stare at a spot on the wall for two to three minutes (feelings of unreality).

- Hyperventilate by breathing deeply and rapidly while sitting down for about one minute (breathlessness, dizziness, numbness or tingling, feelings of unreality).

- Jog in place for two to three minutes or climb stairs for one minute (racing heart, breathlessness)

- Breathe in and out through a small straw for one to two minutes. Hold your nostrils together so you don't breathe through your nose (breathlessness, smothering feelings).

- Stare at a light for one minute and then try to read a book (blurred vision, feelings of unreality).

- Wear extra clothes in a warm room (hot flashes, sweating, racing heart).

- Be creative! If the above exercises don't target sensations that you fear most, invent some ways to produce them.

Exercise	Symptoms	Anxiety (0 to 100)	Similarity (0 to 100)
Shake head			
Hold breath			
Spin in chair			
Stare at wall			
Hyperventilate			
Jog in place/stair climb			
Breathe through straw			
Stare at light			
Wear warm clothes			

When you are finished, take a look at your chart. Circle the five items you found to be most similar to your panic attacks. Now rank those five in order of how much anxiety they caused for you by placing numbers 1 through 5 (with 5 indicating the lowest anxiety) next to the exercise name. As an example, Christine completed these physical symptom exposure exercises after getting clearance from her doctor. Here's how she filled out the chart:

Exercise	Symptoms	Anxiety (0-100)	Similarity (0-100)
② Shake head	Dizzy, unreal	70	60
Hold breath	---	---	---
④ Spin in chair	Nauseated, dizzy	55	55
⑤ Stare at wall	Blurry vision, unreal	50	45
Hyperventilate	---	---	---
① Climb stairs	Breathless, heart pounding, sweating	85	90
Straw breathe	---	---	---
Stare at light	Blurry vision.	40	10
③ Wear warm clothes	Sweaty, heart pounding	60	75

Practicing Physical Symptom Exposure

Now that you've created your hierarchy and you have identified your top five feared sensations, it's time to face those symptoms directly. With repetition, you'll begin to fear those sensations less and less. As is the case with real-life exposures, it is important to practice often—at least once or twice per day. Remember, the more you practice, the faster your anxiety will decrease.

Practice Confronting Feared Sensations

Begin by choosing the lowest-ranked item on your list, and use the following steps to practice confronting your fears:

1. Do the symptom induction activity you chose to bring on the feared sensations.

2. Record your level of anxiety in response to the exercise from 0 to 100.

3. After a few minutes, when the physical symptoms have died down, repeat steps one and two.

4. Continue in this manner until your anxiety is reduced to about half of its starting level. You may have to repeat the exercise several times.

Daily Physical Symptom Exposure Log	Date:
Exercise Practiced:	Anxiety Level (0 to 100)
Trial 1	
Trial 2	
Trial 3	
Trial 4	
Trial 5	
Trial 6	

When the exercise no longer produces much anxiety for you, move on to the next item on your list. Continue until you've worked through all the items on your hierarchy. If you think this sounds hard, you are not alone. Our clients often question the logic of creating the very symptoms they hate *on purpose*. But as long as you continue to be fearful of these uncomfortable, but harmless, physical sensations, you will remain vulnerable to anxiety and panic. Instead, face these symptoms head-on and regain control of your body and your life.

Coping with Other Physical Symptoms During Pregnancy

Not all pregnancy-related physical changes lead to panic, but many can cause worry, anxiety, or discomfort. Use the following tips to cope with these symptoms.

Faintness or Dizziness. It is common for women to experience faintness or dizziness at times during pregnancy, particularly in warm weather or while taking a hot shower. These symptoms are usually due to normal circulatory changes that occur during pregnancy, or they could be a sign of hypoglycemia or anemia; for this reason, it's important to talk with your obstetrician if you have these symptoms. Understandably, these feelings can be disconcerting and lead to anxiety if misinterpreted. In order to lessen the occurrence of these symptoms, try the following tips:

- Take it slowly when changing positions. When sitting or standing up, be more deliberate than usual in order to minimize sudden changes in blood pressure.

- Move more slowly in general. Remember, your body is working especially hard right now. Take breaks and allow more time to get where you're going, particularly when walking.

- Stay cool. Dress in layers and don't get overheated. Take a cool bath or crank up the air conditioner when you need to.

- Eat right. Be sure to drink plenty of fluids and try eating small, healthy snacks throughout the day to avoid major blood sugar fluctuations, which can lead to faintness.

- Exercise. Talk with your doctor about an exercise plan that will work for you. Walking and yoga are two good options.

Fatigue. Pregnancy is exhausting! Your body is working overtime to support your growing baby. Changes in heart rate and blood flow can leave you feeling wiped out—not to mention the accompanying emotional roller-coaster ride filled with excitement, anxiety, anticipation, and fear. Here are some ways you can cope with the fatigue of pregnancy:

- Acknowledge that you need rest. This is a special time in your life when you may not be able to do everything that you usually do. Take naps when you need to and rest up for the important job you and your body are doing.

- Say no. Turn down extra jobs and responsibilities whenever possible. This is not the time to chase down that promotion or remodel the house. Focus your energies on doing only what needs to be done right now.

- Ask for help. It may be difficult to do sometimes, but it's important that you ask for support when you need it. Delegate tasks if you can. You'll find that most people will be more than happy to help you out during this special time.

- Take care of yourself. Be sure to eat a healthy, balanced diet and exercise regularly. Talk to your doctor if you have questions about nutrition or activities that are right for you.

Nausea and Vomiting. The term "morning sickness" is a misnomer, since it is common for women to experience nausea and vomiting around the clock, not just in the morning, particularly in the first trimester; thankfully, it usually subsides by around fourteen weeks. Those first few months can be a frustrating time, when even a whiff of your favorite foods sends you running for the bathroom. During this time, a feedback loop sometimes develops—apprehension or anxiety about vomiting can escalate your nausea, which leads to increased anxiety and then further nausea, and so on. To avoid making your nausea worse by adding anxiety to the mix, try these tips for coping:

- Use the relaxation strategies in chapter 4 to reduce your anxiety and relax your body.

- Get outside when you can. Take a walk or open a window; the fresh air may help to decrease your nausea.

- Eat small meals throughout the day to avoid a stomach that is too full or too empty. Bland foods and complex carbohydrates (such as whole-wheat toast and oatmeal) and proteins (such as cheese and peanut butter) may work best to keep your stomach from turning.

- Check your local drugstore for acupressure wrist bands. Normally used to minimize motion sickness, these simple bands can make a world of difference for some women.

- Remember that your nausea is temporary. Use the strategies in chapter 5 to challenge any catastrophic or dramatic thoughts about your nausea that raise your anxiety.

- If your vomiting is frequent, persistent, or severe talk to your obstetrician about it right away.

Insomnia. Ironically, although pregnancy is a time when you need plenty of rest, many women find it hard to sleep. Vivid dreams or even nightmares are common experiences for pregnant women, and finding a comfortable sleeping position may be difficult, especially as pregnancy progresses. Add to that the pressure on your bladder and frequent trips to the bathroom, and there you are, awake at three o'clock in the morning, staring at the ceiling. Even though pregnancy presents special challenges to getting a good night's sleep, there are some steps you can take to improve your chances of getting those needed z's:

- Use your relaxation exercises. Review the exercises in chapter 4 and use them before you go to sleep and when you find yourself awake at night.

- Don't worry about your dreams. Many women overanalyze the dreams they have during pregnancy, which can lead to anxiety and worry. Your mind and body are just processing your fear and excitement at the prospect of parenthood, not to mention the fluctuating hormones and other physical changes you're undergoing. Try journaling your thoughts and using the techniques described in chapter 5.

- Give yourself some time each night to wind down before bed. Read, take a bath, or do something else you find relaxing.

- Make sure your bedroom is dark and quiet.

- Consider avoiding fluids a couple of hours before bedtime in order to decrease nighttime trips to the bathroom.

- Don't exercise right before bed or drink caffeine after four in the afternoon.

- If you don't fall asleep within about twenty minutes, get up and do something boring or relaxing and then try again. Lying in bed worrying about sleeping never helps you sleep.

Headaches. Early in pregnancy many women experience headaches due to increased blood circulation and hormonal changes. Stress and tension can add to this discomfort and lead to worry and anxiety. If you are concerned about your headaches, talk with your obstetrician for additional recommendations. In the meantime, here are some ways you can manage the headaches that frequently occur during pregnancy:

- Relax. Here's another place where the relaxation exercises you learned in chapter 4 can come in handy. Progressive muscle relaxation may be useful if tension is partially responsible for your headaches.

- Minimize stress. Downsize your schedule and delegate responsibilities to coworkers, friends, and family members whenever possible.

- Get a massage. Many massage therapists offer services specially tailored for expectant moms. This can help to relax the tense muscles that can cause headaches.

- Hydrate. Dehydration is another possible cause of headaches. Be sure to drink plenty of fluids. Talk to your doctor if you are unsure of the guidelines for fluid intake during pregnancy.

- Breathe. Getting outside for some fresh air can sometimes be a remedy. Dry air in office or home environments can contribute to headaches. Find a nice spot outdoors to practice your breathing exercises from chapter 4.

Frequent Urination or Urinary Incontinence. During pregnancy, you will become acquainted with the location of every public bathroom within a fifty-mile radius of your home. Between the increased fluids you are drinking, hormonal changes, anxieties, and your growing baby pressing on your bladder, you may feel an almost constant need to urinate. Sneezing, coughing, and changing position may lead to mild urinary incontinence, which is very common but can be disconcerting or anxiety-provoking nonetheless. You can take the steps below to manage your urges to urinate:

- Urinate often. Be sure to respond to your bladder's signals. Incorporate bathroom breaks in your daily activities.

- Don't worry. Stressing about it won't help. In fact, anxiety can even *increase* the frequency of urinary urges. If you worry about the consequences of urinary frequency or incontinence, use the techniques in chapter 5 to journal and challenge your fears.

- Do Kegel exercises frequently. Kegels can strengthen your pelvic floor and reduce leakage and, as a bonus, they help to prepare you for labor and delivery. You can ask your doctor how to perform Kegels correctly or you can find instructions in most pregnancy books. These techniques can also be beneficial in the postpartum period to help with the temporary urinary incontinence that sometimes follows labor and delivery.

Next Steps

After you've tried all five steps we listed in this chapter, step back for a moment to assess how you feel. Has the frequency of your panic attacks decreased? Are you less anxious in response to your physical sensations? If so, great! You are well on your way to getting your anxiety and panic under control. If you're still feeling more anxious than you would like, you can try going back through the steps again or consult with a therapist. Or, if your anxiety is connected with one of the other problems in this book, like worry or obsessive thoughts, you can go to the chapters on those topics and apply the techniques we've described there as well. Remember, practice is the key. Stick with it—it takes hard work and determination to lessen anxiety, but you can do it!

Key Points

- Pregnancy is a time of dramatic physical changes and new physical sensations. Sometimes these normal physical sensations can lead to anxiety or panic attacks.

- Panic attacks are frightening but harmless. They may be triggered by normal physical changes in pregnancy, like breathlessness, or by postpartum stress.

- Your five-step plan for managing panic attacks includes education, relaxation, challenging anxious thoughts, confronting avoided situations, and facing feared physical sensations.

- Aside from panic, a number of physical symptoms during pregnancy can be influenced by or can lead to worry or anxiety.

- Using the strategies described in this chapter can help you to decrease your panic attacks and lower your anxiety.

CHAPTER 9

Cope with Disturbing Thoughts

Mary is in the kitchen preparing an early-morning bottle for her two-month-old. She holds the fussy infant in her free arm and, as she warms the formula, a terrifying thought strikes her like a bolt of lightning: "What if I put her in the microwave?" Her heart pounds, she begins to sweat, and she quickly runs from the kitchen and wakes her husband to take over their daughter's feeding. Mary is convinced that she must be going crazy; as hard as she tries, she cannot get this thought out of her mind. She starts to avoid being alone with her baby and stops taking her into the kitchen. When she must enter the kitchen, she always says a prayer for her daughter's safety. If she happens to see or think of the microwave while saying this prayer, she feels the urge to repeat the prayer until it feels "right." Mary lies awake at night, panicked that she will act on this terrible thought and harm her daughter.

What Mary doesn't know is that she is experiencing symptoms of obsessive-compulsive disorder (OCD). OCD is an anxiety disorder that affects 2 to 3 percent of the population and is common in pregnant and postpartum women.

In this chapter, you'll learn how to identify symptoms of OCD, challenge any faulty beliefs you have about your thoughts, and change the behaviors that maintain your fear. The cognitive-behavioral strategies discussed in this chapter have been shown to be very effective in treating OCD. Your step-by-step plan for coping with obsessions and compulsions will guide you to reduce fear and avoidance, and reclaim your life and your relationship with your baby.

What Is OCD?

As we noted in chapter 3, OCD consists of obsessions and compulsions. Obsessions are recurrent, intrusive thoughts, images, or impulses that seem senseless but nonetheless cause anxiety or distress. Compulsions are repetitive behaviors or mental acts that the person performs in an effort to decrease the anxiety and distress caused by the obsessions. Mary's obsession is "What if I put my baby in the microwave?" This thought causes her a great deal of anxiety, which she tries to cope with through avoidance and by praying for the safety of her daughter.

OCD in Pregnancy and the Postpartum Period

Research suggests that pregnancy and the postpartum phase can be associated with either the start or worsening of OCD. Studies done in several countries find that, in women with OCD, around 20 percent say that their symptoms started during pregnancy. In addition, up to 50 percent of women with OCD report that their symptoms worsened during pregnancy or the postpartum period (Labad et al. 2005; Vulink et al. 2006). In obstetrical clinics, 3.5 percent of women in their third trimester of pregnancy and 4 percent at six weeks postpartum met criteria for OCD (Uguz, Akman, et al. 2007; Uguz, Gezginc, et al. 2007).

The obsessive thoughts of new and expectant mothers tend to be focused on the baby, and often of harm coming to the baby, and these are not restricted to women with OCD. In fact, in a recent study, 100 percent of postpartum women said they had intrusive thoughts of accidental harm coming to their infants—things like suffocation, illness, abduction, or falls (Fairbrother and Woody 2008). Around half of the women also reported intrusive thoughts about intentionally harming their children by shaking, stabbing, drowning, smothering, or sexually molesting them. In pregnancy, thoughts may revolve around fears of contamination, birth defects, or miscarriage. Compulsions in pregnant and postpartum women often include washing and cleaning rituals, compulsive checking, or avoidance.

Women with a family history of OCD seem to be more vulnerable to developing symptoms. In addition, in many cases, symptoms of OCD begin or worsen suddenly within a few weeks after delivery. Unfortunately, women are often reluctant to seek help for this treatable condition for fear that others will not understand, that they will frighten loved ones, or that their children will be taken away.

> ### ~ COMMON QUESTION ~
>
> **If I have these kinds of thoughts, does that mean I have OCD?**
>
> Not necessarily. As you will learn in the following sections, almost everyone has unwanted thoughts from time to time. In fact, thoughts of harm coming to the fetus or newborn frequently happen among women without OCD. However, if these thoughts get in the way of your life or occupy more than one hour of your day then you may be suffering from OCD. Regardless of whether you have OCD or not, the treatment steps outlined in this chapter will be helpful to you.

Obsessions vs. Postpartum Psychosis

While these thoughts can be disturbing, mothers with OCD are unlikely to cause harm to their child. The terrible news stories we see about mothers taking their children's lives are usually associated with severe postpartum depression or psychosis, *not* OCD. Thankfully, postpartum psychosis is extremely rare, occurring in only one or two in every thousand postpartum women (Kendell, Chalmers, and Platz 1987). The chart on the next page highlights the difference between this condition and OCD. If you have any symptoms of postpartum psychosis, contact a medical professional immediately.

OCD	Psychosis
Intrusive thoughts that cause distress	Aggressive thoughts without guilt or distress
Anxiety	Confusion, agitation
Fear of acting on or thinking the thought	Hearing voices or seeing things that other people don't see
Avoidance or rituals	Bizarre or violent behavior

Identifying Your OCD Symptoms

As always, the first step in tackling obsessions and compulsions is to know your symptoms. Below we've listed some common thoughts that pregnant women or new moms have and rituals that they perform. Begin by placing a check mark next to the symptoms that you experience. Don't be worried if you don't see your particular thoughts or behaviors on the list—there are literally endless possibilities and we've left room for you to write in any that you don't see listed.

Obsessions

Contamination Obsessions

I worry excessively that

☐ my baby will get sick from dirt, germs, or bodily secretions

☐ I will come into contact with environmental contaminants (such as lead, mercury, or radon) that will harm my unborn baby

☐ my baby will get a disease like AIDS or hepatitis

☐ household cleansers or chemicals will hurt my unborn baby

☐ my child will get sick from contact with animals or insects

☐ I will contract lysteria or another disease that could harm my unborn baby

☐ Other: _____

☐ Other:_____

Harming Obsessions

I can't stop thinking about

☐ my baby being accidentally harmed by my carelessness

☐ horrific images of harm coming to my baby

☐ harming my baby by acting on an unwanted impulse like drowning, stabbing, or smothering

☐ my baby dying of SIDS or another illness

☐ someone stealing or harming my baby

☐ Other:_____

☐ Other:_____

Sexual Obsessions

I have unwanted intrusive thoughts about

☐ accidentally touching my child inappropriately

☐ images of my baby's genitals

☐ acting on an impulse to molest my own or other children

☐ Other: _____

☐ Other: _____

Other Obsessions

I have other obsessions, including the following:

☐ _____

☐ _____

☐ _____

☐ _____

Compulsions

Cleaning and Washing Compulsions

I excessively, repeatedly, or uncontrollably

☐ sterilize my baby's bottles or pacifiers

☐ wash my hands before touching my baby

☐ bathe or wash my baby

☐ clean the house, floor, or other areas that my baby will touch

☐ disinfect my child's toys or other belongings

☐ avoid people, objects, or places that seem contaminated

☐ Other: _____

☐ Other: _____

Checking Compulsions

I repeatedly check

☐ that my baby is breathing

☐ for evidence of lead, radon, or other contaminants in my home

☐ that my baby is properly secured in his stroller or car seat

☐ that windows and doors are locked and appliances are off

☐ my child's toys for loose parts

☐ for signs that my baby has been abused or injured

☐ Other: _____

☐ Other: _____

Other Compulsions

I perform other compulsions, such as

☐ mental rituals like prayers or repeating "good" thoughts to counter "bad" ones

☐ repeatedly seeking reassurance from others (such as a doctor, significant other, or friend)

☐ avoiding being alone with my baby or child

☐ Other:_____

☐ Other:_____

Your Four-Step Plan to Tackle Obsessions and Compulsions

Now that you know how common symptoms of OCD are during pregnancy and the postpartum period and you've identified which obsessions and compulsions you experience, you're ready to use the skills you learned in part 2 of this book. In this section, we'll describe four key steps to coping with disturbing thoughts during pregnancy or in the postpartum period:

1. Understand your obsessions and compulsions.

2. Challenge your beliefs about your intrusive thoughts.

3. Change unhealthy coping strategies that contribute to anxiety.

4. Confront your feared thoughts and situations.

Step One: Understanding Your Obsessions and Compulsions

One of the common concerns we hear from our clients is that it is "not normal" to have such terrible thoughts. This is simply not true. Although you may feel as if you are alone in dealing with these painful thoughts, you are not. Researchers around the world have found that up to 90 percent of the population experience unwanted intrusive thoughts. In postpartum women *without* OCD, repetitive thoughts of harming their children (either by accident or intentionally), of accidents, of sexual misconduct, and of infant death frequently occur (Abramowitz, Schwartz, Moore, and Luenzmann 2003). Ask a friend, a relative, or your doctor if she has ever had an intrusive thought—if the person is being honest, she will tell you that she has.

So, if everyone has these thoughts, why are they so frequent, intense, and distressing for some women? The answer lies in how you *respond* to the thoughts. When most people have an intrusive thought, they hardly notice it and, if they do, they are able to easily dismiss it. What allows that thought to become stuck and cause anxiety is the belief that the thought is important, dangerous, or meaningful in some way (Salkovskis 1999). For instance, if Mary believes that her thought "What if I put my baby in the microwave?" means that she is evil or crazy and that she may act on the thought, then it will cause her great anxiety. In an attempt to decrease this anxiety, she develops avoidance strategies (like never being alone with her baby) or rituals to "prevent" the action from occurring (like praying for her baby's safety). Unfortunately, instead of decreasing anxiety, these strategies actually cause Mary to be even more vigilant against the thoughts and they themselves become triggers for the obsessions. In this way, the cycle of obsessions and compulsions perpetuates itself.

Our clients often ask, "Why can't I just stop thinking about it?!" These thoughts are terribly disturbing, particularly for new moms or moms-to-be, and of course you'd like to just wipe them from your mind. New parents often use strategies like distraction or avoidance to combat their intrusive thoughts, but these methods are rarely successful in the long term. With our own clients, we use the exercise below to illustrate just how impossible it is to intentionally *not* think about something. Try it for yourself and see how well you do.

Exercise: Don't Think of a Red Balloon

Find an egg timer or a watch with an alarm and set it to ring after one minute. Close your eyes and think about whatever you'd like, but do *not* think of a red balloon. Don't think of the word "balloon" and certainly don't allow an image of a balloon to come into your mind! Stick with it for a full minute and count how many times you slip up and allow thoughts or images of the balloon to enter your mind.

How did you do? If you're like most people, you probably weren't very successful at all; the more you tried to not think about it, the more the balloon tended to pop into your mind. In fact, some researchers have found the same thing: the more we try to suppress thoughts, the more likely they are to occur (Wegman 1994). And even when people can manage to do it, they find it difficult to maintain this level of concentration for very long.

So, now that you understand what obsessions and compulsions are, how they function together to cause anxiety, and why your current coping strategies don't work, you are ready to learn some new ways to deal with these thoughts.

Step Two: Challenging Your Beliefs About Obsessions

The second step in tackling intrusive thoughts or obsessions is to challenge your beliefs about them. In chapter 5, you learned how to evaluate and counter your anxious thoughts. With some slight modification, you can use this technique to decrease your anxiety related to obsessions as well. Women who experience disturbing thoughts about their children are often worried that having these thoughts means something terrible about them, like that they are dangerous or violent or that they don't actually care for or love their children. Ironically, the opposite is true—the thoughts that cause you the most distress are the ones about what is *most* important to you. This is just one of the many ways that women can misinterpret their thoughts.

Common Misinterpretations of Intrusive Thoughts

Below we have listed some of the more common beliefs about your thoughts that can lead to anxiety and start that cycle of obsessions and compulsions spinning.

Overestimation of Risk, Threat, or Importance. Some women may have a tendency to think that a particular thought is important. They may overestimate the importance of an obsession or the likelihood or the severity of negative consequences. If this is true for you, you may think the following:

- "If I have a thought about hurting my baby, it means I may act on it."

- "Only evil or crazy people have these kinds of thoughts."

> ### ~ COMMON QUESTION ~
> #### How do these beliefs contribute to my anxiety?
>
> It is no surprise that, if you believe they are significant, meaningful, or dangerous, you will be distressed by intrusive thoughts. Remember, though, that almost *everyone* has bad, intrusive thoughts. If you view these thoughts accurately, as the normal and inconsequential musings of your mind, you are unlikely to be anxious and will be able to dismiss them more easily. If, on the other hand, you subscribe to the beliefs listed, anxiety is sure to follow.

Exaggerated Responsibility. Postpartum or pregnant women may believe that if they can have any influence over a negative outcome then they are responsible for preventing it, no matter how small the probability of its occurrence. You might believe the following:

- "I must vigilantly guard against making any mistake that could possibly cause harm to my child, no matter how remote the chances are."

- "Even a tiny chance of something bad happening still requires me to act."

Need for Certainty or Perfection. Perhaps you believe that you need total certainty about the occurrence of a bad event in order to feel comfortable, or you may believe that there is one perfect way of doing things that will make everything okay:

- "If I cannot prove that I will definitely not molest my child, I won't be able to stand it."

- "Because I sometimes have bad thoughts about my baby, my love for him is forever tainted."

Thought-Action Fusion. You may believe that thinking about a negative event actually increases its likelihood of happening, or that thinking bad thoughts is the same as acting on them:

- "If I have a thought of harming my child, I feel as if I've actually done it."

- "When I worry about my baby dying of SIDS, I feel it may jinx her and cause it to happen."

Need for Control over Thoughts. Women in pregnancy or the postpartum period may feel the need to have perfect control over their intrusive thoughts in order to maintain control over their behavior. If you feel this way, you may think the following:

- "If I don't keep these thoughts out of my mind, I may snap and go crazy."

- "Because I can't stop these thoughts, it must mean something terrible about me."

Changing Your Beliefs About Your Intrusive Thoughts

Now it's time to challenge those misinterpretations and lower your anxiety. In chapter 5, we described several techniques for changing your thinking. Remember, in this case, you are trying to change your *beliefs* about the obsessions or intrusive thoughts, not the thoughts themselves. Arguing with the thought will usually get you nowhere. Consider what happens when Mary gets into a mental debate with her intrusive thought:

OCD: What if you put your baby in the microwave?

Mary: Oh my God, I would never do that. I love my baby.

OCD: Are you sure? Why would you have a thought like that if you didn't want to act on it?

Mary: That's true, I don't know for sure. It can't be normal to think this way. Maybe I really am dangerous. I should stay away from my baby.

OCD: Right!

As you can see, arguing with your obsessive thoughts is futile. In fact, engaging in a debate with your obsessions often makes your anxiety worse, because it makes these thoughts seem important and meaningful. By changing how you view your obsessive thoughts, you can take the sting out of them and stop fighting the losing battle of arguing logic with an irrational opponent.

Mary used a modified version of a thought record to change her beliefs about her intrusive thoughts instead of arguing directly with them.

Mary's Intrusive Thought Worksheet

Date	Intrusive Thought	Belief (0 to 100)	Emotions (0 to 100)	Balanced Response	Outcome (Rerate belief and emotion 0 to 100)
July 12	Image of my baby in the microwave	What kind of mother am I? I wouldn't be having thoughts like this unless part of me wanted to harm my baby. If I can't stop thinking like this, I may really hurt my daughter. I must be crazy. Belief: 90	Fear: 95 Guilt: 90 Sadness: 75	I have generally shown that I am a good mother and I don't feel like I want to harm my child. In fact, I'm very upset about the idea. There is a big difference between having these thoughts and acting on them. I have many thoughts that I don't act on. I know now that almost every mother has these kinds of scary thoughts, so it doesn't mean I'm crazy.	Fear: 70 Guilt: 50 Sadness: 40 Belief: 60

Another example comes from Valerie. She is pregnant and has obsessive thoughts that her unborn baby may be harmed by environmental contaminants, germs, or diseases. As a result, she washes and cleans excessively and avoids strangers and public places. Her thought record is on the following page.

			Valerie's Intrusive Thought Worksheet		
Date	**Intrusive Thought**	**Belief (0 to 100)**	**Emotions (0 to 100)**	**Balanced Response**	**Outcome (Rerate belief and emotion 0 to 100)**
May 7	What if that cheese I ate earlier wasn't pasteurized like I thought it was?	I can't believe I am so careless. I shouldn't have done that without being completely certain. That's as bad intentionally putting the baby in harm's way. Belief: 80	Fear: 80 Guilt: 95 Anxiety: 75	There is a possibility that I was wrong about the cheese being pasteurized, but it is a pretty small chance. I am more careful than most of my friends are and all their babies have been fine. If I did make a mistake, that is not really the same as hurting the baby on purpose.	Fear: 30 Guilt: 40 Anxiety: 25 Belief: 40

Now it's your turn! Make copies of the form on the following page or record the information in a notebook or journal. Pick a recent intrusive thought that you have experienced and use the following questions to help you challenge your beliefs about your thought:

- Am I making any of the misinterpretations discussed earlier in this chapter?

- What is the evidence for and against this belief?

- Are there any other possibilities?

- Is this a fact or an opinion?

- What would I say to a friend if she told me this about herself?

- Is this very realistic or likely to come true?

Intrusive Thought Worksheet

Date	Intrusive Thought	Belief (0 to 100)	Emotions (0 to 100)	Balanced Response	Outcome (Rerate belief and emotion 0 to 100)

Exercise: Challenge Your Beliefs About Your Intrusive Thoughts

After you have practiced countering your beliefs about one of your previous thoughts, you may now try to use this method as your thoughts arise. Don't worry if it is hard at first. Keep at it and it will get easier. Practice challenging your beliefs at least once every day. Eventually you will be able to do it without even writing anything down.

Step Three: Change Your Unhealthy Coping Strategies

As we emphasized in chapter 6, an important step in beating your obsessions and compulsions is *response prevention*. When you are doing the exposures coming up in step four, it is critical that you resist the urge to use your usual coping strategies or rituals. Some of the most common unhealthy coping strategies among pregnant and new moms include excessive cleaning and washing, checking, and mental rituals as well as avoidance and reassurance seeking. In our clinical practice, we find that rituals like checking and cleaning and washing tend to be fairly obvious. The mental rituals, reassurance seeking, and avoidance are trickier to identify and tackle. These can masquerade as normal, reasonable actions that many moms might take. Remember, though, that if you are performing these thoughts or actions in order to decrease anxiety about your obsessions, then they are compulsions. Look for these clues that your behavior may be a ritual that is feeding your anxiety:

- Do you frequently respond to bad thoughts with good ones or with prayer?

- Do you find yourself arguing with your intrusive thoughts?

- Do you doubt yourself, or do have trouble making decisions without asking the opinion of others?

- Do you repeatedly ask your spouse, family, friends, or doctors the same questions?

- Do you consistently avoid certain situations or objects?

- Do you avoid being alone with your baby?

If you answered yes to any of these questions, add the behaviors to the table on the next page:

My Maladaptive Coping Strategies or Rituals
(Excessive Cleaning, Checking, Avoidance, Mental Rituals, or Reassurance Seeking)

Step Four: Confront Feared Thoughts and Situations

In chapter 6, we discussed exposure therapy and how helpful it can be for anxiety problems. Many researchers have studied exposure therapy in people with obsessions and compulsions, and they've consistently found it to be extremely helpful for as many as 80 percent of those who try it. In this step, you will learn how to apply both real life and imaginal exposures to confront the thoughts and situations that you have been avoiding.

Using Exposure to Master Your Obsessions

One of the main reasons for using exposure is to learn that your fearful predictions just aren't true. By repeatedly exposing yourself to your obsessive thoughts and anxiety-provoking situations without using your usual coping strategies, you will see that your anxiety goes down, that the disturbing thoughts become less frequent, and that your fears don't come true.

In order for exposure therapy to be effective, though, remember that you need to be anxious during the exposures and stick with the exposure until your anxiety diminishes. Refrain from any behaviors or thoughts that reduce your anxiety during exposures, even though the urge may be strong. Remember, your anxiety will decrease on its own without your doing anything at all to lower it, and by refraining from responding to it, you will be learning that you do not need to fear it.

Your Exposure Hierarchy. Look back at your exposure hierarchy in chapter 6 or, if you haven't yet created one, use the instructions there to make a list of your feared thoughts or situations. Make sure to put any situations or thoughts on it that you avoid. Remember to list your items in order of how much anxiety you would feel if you confronted them without your usual coping strategies or rituals, with 100 representing the worst anxiety you can imagine, 0 meaning no anxiety, and 50 indicating moderate anxiety.

Below is an example of Valerie's exposure hierarchy.

Feared Thoughts, Objects, and Situations	Anxiety
Eating at a party or restaurant where I don't know every ingredient included in the food.	100
Being on the commuter train during rush hour	95
Putting gasoline in my car	85
Shaking hands with a client at work	85
Eating lunch at the house of a friend who has a cat	75
Using a public bathroom	70
Eating nonorganic vegetables	60
Using nail polish	55
Sitting near the computer	50

Now, create your own exposure hierarchy, below.

Feared Thoughts, Objects, and Situations	Anxiety

Now that you've completed your hierarchy, select an item low on the list—something challenging but not overwhelming. Practice exposing yourself to that situation and try to stay with it until your anxiety diminishes by about half. How long this takes varies from person to person—it may take twenty minutes or it may take an hour. But it is important that you don't quit before your anxiety decreases. If you are a new mom and your baby doesn't always want to wait for you to habituate before you change or feed her, try to pick exposures that you can do repeatedly throughout the day rather than ones that require long stretches of time. Examples of this type of exposure on Valerie's hierarchy might be shaking hands with someone, using a public bathroom, and eating nonorganic vegetables.

Make copies of the form below so you can use it to rate your anxiety during the exposure exercise and see your progress over time. When an exposure causes you only mild or no anxiety, it is time to move up to the next item on your hierarchy and repeat the process. Continue to confront your fears until you have completed all the items on your list. If you have questions regarding the safety of any exposures, be sure to ask your doctor. For example, when Valerie started, she rated sitting near the computer at an anxiety level of 50. She stayed near the computer that first day until her anxiety decreased to level of 25. Each day that week, she sat near the computer until, after a few days, it no longer caused her much anxiety. She then moved to the next item on her list and continued this way until she had addressed all the items on her hierarchy. If you are having any trouble with the process or your anxiety is not decreasing, look back at the tips for successful exposures listed near the end of chapter 6.

Exposure Practice Form
Date: _____
Exposure to practice: _____
Rituals to prevent: _____
_____
_____
Start time: _____ End time: _____
Anxiety level (0 to 100):
Start: _____ Notes: _____
10 minutes: _____ _____
20 minutes: _____ _____
30 minutes: _____ _____
40 minutes: _____ _____
50 minutes: _____ _____
60 minutes: _____ _____
End: _____ _____

Confronting Feared Thoughts

Many times, items on your list may not be situations or objects to which you can easily expose yourself to in real life. In fact, during pregnancy or the postpartum phase, *thoughts* themselves are often the feared stimulus. Remember Mary? She was experiencing intrusive thoughts of putting her baby in the microwave. Her hierarchy looked like this:

Feared Thoughts, Objects, and Situations	Anxiety
The thought or image of my baby in the microwave	100
Holding my baby while using the microwave	95
Being in the kitchen alone with my baby	90
Looking at the microwave	85
Being in the house alone with my baby	75
Thinking of the microwave while looking at my baby's picture	70
Holding my baby when someone else is home	60
Thinking the word "microwave" along with my baby's name	55
Eating dinner in the kitchen with my husband present	40

Mary addressed some items on her hierarchy in the same way that Valerie did, by confronting the situation directly. She started out by eating dinner in the kitchen with her husband each night until her anxiety diminished. However, some items on her list are not feared situations or objects but feared *thoughts*. Mary addressed those using the imaginal exposure technique we described in chapter 6—in which the exposures take place in one's imagination. For instance, the top item on Mary's hierarchy is the thought or image of her baby in the microwave. Mary used imaginal exposure to confront this feared thought using the steps below:

1. Choose a thought from your hierarchy.

2. Write a detailed story about the thought and your most feared consequences of that thought.

3. Record the story using an audiotape or digital recorder.

4. Listen to the story repeatedly until your anxiety decreases.

Mary's imaginal script looked something like this:

My husband is away at a business dinner and I am using the microwave to heat some leftovers for my dinner. I am holding my fussy baby and I am so exhausted that I can barely see straight. The microwave beeps to signal my dinner is ready and by now my baby is crying loudly so I know that I, once more, will not get to eat anything. Like a zombie, I remove my food and replace it with my baby. She looks up at me with her big eyes, looking confused and scared about what is happening. With no one home to stop me, I shut the door, turn it on, and walk away. I can hear her muffled screams from the next room but I do nothing. When my husband returns home to this grisly scene he is out of his mind with grief. I am taken away by the police. After the trial, my husband divorces me and my parents cannot bear to talk to me. Completely alone, I spend the rest of my days in an institution for the criminally insane, thinking about how I killed my innocent child and ruined the lives of everyone I love.

After writing out this scene, Mary recorded it onto an audiotape and listened to it each day. In each of her exposure sessions, she repeatedly listened to the story while imagining the scenario as vividly as possible. This was extremely difficult for her at first. She reported that her anxiety level was 100, and that she was tearful and distressed as she visualized this terrible scene. But, over time, the tears stopped and her anxiety decreased. And something amazing happened—she noticed that she was having fewer of these thoughts and that she wasn't so anxious when a thought did pop into her head. She began to enjoy the time she spent with her daughter instead of dreading it. She reclaimed her life and her relationship with her baby.

But This Sounds Terrible! Of course, if something bad happened to your baby, it would be awful. It is a sad thing when someone we love is hurt. But the important distinction to make here is that the *thought* of something bad happening is not the same as something bad *actually* happening. These thoughts can be so scary that they can seem like the same thing, but they are not. Through exposure, you will begin to tolerate the occurrence of these normal, although frightening thoughts, and see for yourself that having the thought does not lead to the thing you fear.

Next Steps

After you've tried all four steps we listed in this chapter, take a moment to see how you feel. Has the frequency of your intrusive thoughts decreased? Are you less anxious in response to them? Have you stopped avoiding the thoughts or situations? If your answer is yes, that's wonderful! You are on the way to getting your life back. If you're still having trouble, you can try going back through the steps again or consult a cognitive-behavioral therapist in your area. If your anxiety is partially based on one of the other problems in this book, like panic or worry, try going to the chapters on that specific problem and apply the techniques we've described there. Remember, though, with exposure therapy, practice and repetition are the keys. Stick with it—over time you should see your anxiety decrease.

Key Points

➻ Disturbing obsessions, or intrusive thoughts, are common in pregnancy and the post-partum phase and almost everyone has these kinds of "bad" thoughts at one time or another.

➻ How you respond to the thoughts determines their frequency and how much anxiety you experience in relation to them.

➻ Understanding these thoughts thoroughly and challenging your beliefs about them is an important step in decreasing your anxiety.

➻ Confronting your fears *without* using unhealthy coping strategies has been shown to be a very effective treatment for obsessions and compulsions.

➻ With practice, you can change your reaction to these thoughts, lower your anxiety, and reclaim your relationship with your baby.

CHAPTER 10

Conquer Worry

Are you a worrier? If so, you're not alone—almost everyone worries at times, and many people consider themselves worriers. As you might expect, parenthood can be a particularly challenging time for those who tend to worry. After all, there is an endless list of possible worries for moms and moms-to-be: Will my baby be healthy? Will I be a good mom? Will my marriage survive? Will I still have a life?

Most of the time, worry isn't much of an issue. In fact, productive worry can actually spur us on to take action and solve our problems. For instance, worrying that you need to find a good pediatrician for your soon-to-arrive baby may push you to research your options and make a decision well before your due date. However, when worry is unproductive, excessive, and out of control, it can cause physical symptoms such as headaches, backaches, nausea, and insomnia. Chronic worry can also damage your relationships and make other problems, such as depression and procrastination, worse.

The good news is that you can learn to control worry. In this chapter, we'll show you five key techniques you can use to defeat worry for good. This step-by-step plan will help you turn your worry around so you can relax and enjoy the wonders of being a mom.

What Is Worry?

"Worry" is a term that gets thrown around a lot, but it can be surprisingly difficult to define. Even therapists and researchers disagree at times about what "worry" means. For our purposes, we define "worry" as *catastrophic thinking*, which is *focused on the future*.

Melissa's thoughts provide a good example of worry. Melissa was four months pregnant when she started therapy for anxiety. During one session, she tearfully described her worst fears:

- That her baby would develop autism in childhood

- That she wouldn't be able to handle having a child with special needs

- That she'd go broke paying for doctors and therapists and get divorced

Let's examine these three thoughts in more detail. Melissa is clearly thinking about the *future* when she worries that her baby might develop autism. She's also thinking in *catastrophic* terms when she tells herself "I won't be able to handle it" and when she predicts that she'll go broke and get divorced. When we look at these thoughts closely, we can see that they fit our definition of worry— thinking catastrophically about the future.

Worry in Pregnancy and the Postpartum Period

Perhaps not surprisingly, in light of the stress of caring for a baby, studies have found that rates of excessive worry are higher in postpartum women than they are in the general population. Around 8 percent of postpartum women in one study indicated that they suffered clinically significant symptoms of worry. In addition, many women who worried frequently before becoming pregnant found that their worry got worse after the birth of their child (Wenzel et al. 2005). Unfortunately, little research has been done that looks specifically at worry during pregnancy and the postpartum period. However, worry in general has been studied extensively, leading to the development of clinically proven strategies to manage worry. You can use these same methods to control your worry. In this section, you'll learn to identify the things you worry about most often. Then, you'll learn specific strategies to bring your worry under control.

Common Worries You Might Experience

In our work with anxious moms and moms-to-be, we've noticed that the most common worries of new moms usually fall into one of four categories: (1) labor and delivery, (2) your baby's health, (3) your competence as a mother, and (4) the impact of a baby on your life.

Let's take a look at some examples of common worries for each of these categories.

Labor and Delivery

- *I won't be able to handle the pain.*
- *I won't know what to do.*
- *Something could go wrong.*
- *What if I can't do it?*

Your Baby's Health

- *What if my baby has a birth defect or medical condition like cerebral palsy?*
- *What if our house or toys contain lead paint?*
- *What if my baby dies of SIDS?*
- *What if the plastic in my son's bottles makes him sick?*

Your Competence as a Mother

- *What if I don't have a maternal instinct?*
- *What if I'm a terrible mother?*
- *I'll never be able to do this.*
- *What if I make the same mistakes my mom made?*

The Impact of a Baby on Your Life

- *I'll never see my friends again.*
- *Our marriage will be ruined.*
- *We won't be able to travel or do fun things.*
- *I'll never lose this baby weight.*

> ### ~ COMMON QUESTION ~
> #### What if my worries don't fall into these categories?
>
> If some of the things you worry about don't fall neatly into these categories, don't be concerned. New moms and moms-to-be can have a variety of worries—the options are nearly limitless. The things you worry about are as unique as your baby's little footprint. Regardless of your specific worries, the five-step plan in this chapter is effective for any type of worry.

Think about the things you've worried about over the past week or two. Did any of them fall into these categories? For example, did you have any concerns about your baby's health? Did you worry at all about your mothering skills? Were you anxious about labor and delivery? Starting to identify common themes in your worry can be a useful step toward defeating it. In the next section, you'll learn how to track your worry using a worry diary. Keeping a worry diary will help you pinpoint the things you worry about the most.

Tracking Your Worries

Before you start working directly on controlling your worry, you might find it helpful to use a worry diary to track your worries for a week or so. This activity can have two key benefits. First, you can evaluate your thoughts to see if they are actual worries. Second, you can pinpoint which of the four areas of worry you struggle with the most.

Let's take a look at Leslie's worry diary. Leslie was about three months pregnant with her first child when she started therapy for anxiety. Here's a sample of the worries that Leslie recorded over the course of a week.

Leslie's Worry Diary		
Date/Time	**Situation**	**Worry**
August 9 9:00 a.m.	Watching a tuna commercial	Oh my God. I ate tuna that one time! I didn't know I wasn't supposed to. What if it had mercury? What if I caused my child to have a birth defect?
August 9 8:00 p.m.	Talking with my husband about possible names	The other kids will pick on our child. He'll be made fun of and bullied all through school.
August 10 1:15 p.m.	Reading a magazine article on the cost of raising a child	We're never going to able to afford all this stuff. We're going to go broke.
August 11 7:30 a.m.	Driving	I need to get a car seat. What if we don't get one installed before our baby is born? Then we'll be scrambling at the last minute and we'll have so many other things to do.
August 11 12:30 p.m.	Driving	What if we're driving home from the hospital with the baby and we have an accident?"
August 11 4:30 P.M.	Seeing a mom who looked all stressed out at the mall	What if I can't handle being a mom? What if I'm a terrible mother?
August 12 11:30 A.M.	Planning a weekend getaway with friends	This is the last time I'll ever get to do this. I'll probably hardly ever see my friends again.
August 12 2:00 P.M.	Having lunch with a friend who has two kids	She's such a good mom. I'll never be that good. My kids will grow up with all kinds of problems because of me.

After looking at Leslie's worry diary, ask yourself this question: Is Leslie actually worrying? Even though Leslie listed these thoughts in her worry diary, they might not be worries. So let's put them to the test to find out if they truly are worries. Remember, worry has two key elements: (1) it always involves catastrophic thoughts, and (2) those thoughts are about the future.

Do any of Leslie's thoughts fit these criteria? Let's look at the components of worry one at a time. First, is Leslie thinking catastrophically? As you look at her thoughts closely, you'll see that Leslie is thinking about the process of becoming a mom in the worst possible light. Her image of motherhood is filled with challenges, threats, failures, and isolation. Leslie's thoughts are clear examples of catastrophic thinking.

How about our second criterion? Is Leslie thinking about the future? One sign of thinking about the future is the presence of "what if" thoughts. Leslie has listed several "what if" thoughts in her worry diary. For example, she recorded thoughts such as "What if we get into a car accident?" and "What if I'm a terrible mother?" That tells us she's thinking about things that haven't happened yet—the future—so these thoughts meet our second criterion. In other words, Leslie is worrying.

Now that we know Leslie is worrying, let's see if her thoughts fit into any of the common categories of worry. Take a look at her first worry. She's thinking, "What if the tuna I ate had mercury in it?" and "What if that causes a birth defect?" Which of the four categories listed above do you think this worry fits into?

If you said "baby's health" you're correct. Leslie is clearly worrying about her baby's health because she's worried that her child will be born with a birth defect.

What other types of worry does Leslie have? Put your answers in the space below:

_____

_____

_____

_____

If you answered that Leslie is also worrying about her competence as a mother and the impact of having a baby on her life, congratulations—you are correct! Nice work. After reviewing Leslie's worry diary, we can see that Leslie is worried that her baby won't be healthy, she won't be a good mother, and she'll never have time for friends.

Now it's your turn to give worry tracking a try. Use the worry diary form to track your worries for one week. Keep in mind that, like Leslie, you will probably record worries from more than one category.

Exercise: Keep a Worry Diary

For the next week, keep track of your worries using the worry diary form that follows. Note the time, date, situation, and what you were worried about. Be specific. Note exactly what was going through your mind.

My Worry Diary		
Date/Time	Situation	Worry

After tracking your worries for a week or so, take a look at your worry diary. First, check your worries to make sure that they are actually worries. As you'll recall, you can identify a worry by the fact that it involves catastrophic thinking about the future. Remember, even though it's called a "worry diary," some of the thoughts you record might not meet the definition of a worry.

Now take a look at the worries you recorded in your diary. Which of the four areas of worry did you engage in? Make a check mark below next to any that applied to you:

☐ Labor and delivery

☐ Your baby's health

☐ Your competence as a mother

☐ The impact of a baby on your life

You might've also found that you worried about one area more than others. Circle that one. You'll want to pay special attention to that theme as you work through the next section.

Your Five-Step Plan for Conquering Worry

Now that you understand what worry is and you've gotten a feel for your own worries by tracking them, you're ready to learn how to take charge of your worry and keep it from controlling your life. In this section, we'll describe five key steps to defeating worry:

1. Practice relaxation.

2. Determine whether your worry is productive.

3. Change your thoughts.

4. Use exposure and response prevention.

5. Accept uncertainty.

Step One: Practice Relaxation

The first step in your plan for overcoming worry is to master the ability to deeply relax. As you learned in chapter 4, deep relaxation is a skill, which you need to practice in order to master. Unfortunately, chronic worry erodes that skill, leaving you in a constant state of high alert. Worse yet, the constant arousal of your nervous system can also lead to unpleasant physical symptoms, such as the following:

• muscle tension

• difficulty concentrating

• restlessness

• fatigue

- insomnia

- shaking

- sweating

- lightheadedness

- nausea

- diarrhea

In chapter 4, you learned three relaxation techniques for countering the effects of anxiety and stress: diaphragmatic breathing, progressive muscle relaxation, and guided imagery. For those who suffer from chronic worry, these techniques are crucial to managing the physical symptoms that comes with worry.

Exercise: Practice Relaxation

Recall the relaxation techniques you practiced in chapter 4. Which relaxation technique worked best for you? In our clinical practices, we find that PMR works particularly well for worry, but you may find that another strategy is more effective for you. Continue to practice that technique each day for about twenty minutes.

More Ways You Can Relax

Cultivating the ability to deeply relax doesn't need to be confined to twenty minutes of daily practice with a specific technique. In fact, the more times each day you experience a sense of calmness and peace, the better. Here are other ways to relax:

- Massage

- Yoga

- Reading

- Gardening

- Scrapbooking

- Exercise

- Taking a warm bath

- Painting

- Playing a musical instrument

- Watching a movie

- Talking to a friend

- Listening to music

- Other activities you find relaxing: _____

_____

Exercise: Schedule Relaxing Activities

Take a look at the list above. Which activities sound relaxing and enjoyable to you? Be sure to engage in those activities as frequently as possible to counter the effects of excessive worry.

Step Two: Determine if Your Worry Is Productive

As you learned in chapter 7, all worry is not created equal; in fact, there are two types of worry: *productive worry* and *unproductive worry*. Determining whether your worry is productive or unproductive is a key step in controlling it and it helps you decide which strategies will be most helpful.

Defining Productive vs. Unproductive Worry

Let's review the three key features of productive worry:

- It's focused on the present or immediate future.

- The problem is specific and likely to occur.

- There are definite steps you can take to solve the problem.

Unproductive worry, on the other hand, meets the following criteria:

- It is focused on the more distant future.

- The problem is unlikely; it has a low probability of occurring.

- The problem is unsolvable or the power to change it is out of your control.

To see the difference in these two types of worry, let's look back at Leslie's worry diary. The first item that Leslie listed was focused on some tuna she ate while pregnant. This is an unproductive worry since the consequences would occur in the distant future, there's a low probability that her child's health would suffer, and, other than avoiding tuna in the future, there's nothing Leslie can do now to eliminate the risk, however low.

Now, let's look at the first worry Leslie had while driving—she was worrying about getting a car seat. This is a good example of a productive worry. Although this worry is targeted at the more distant future, since she's just three months pregnant, it is a specific concern, and there are definite steps Leslie can take to solve this problem. To resolve this worry, Leslie simply needs to get a car seat and install it.

Coping with Productive Worry

As you might conclude, one of the best ways you can cope with your productive worry is to solve the problem. (Recall chapter 7, where you learned problem solving as a key technique that you can apply to productive worries.) If you've analyzed a worry and determined that it is productive, use the problem-solving techniques in chapter 7 to defeat your worry.

Managing Unproductive Worry

Unproductive worry, of course, is a bit more difficult to deal with—you can't just solve the problem that's worrying you. We focus on controlling unproductive worry in this chapter. The next three steps will guide you through therapeutic techniques to help you conquer unproductive worry.

Exercise: Is Your Worry Productive or Unproductive?

Now is a good time to take a look at your worry diary and identify productive and unproductive worries. Look at each worry you have recorded over the past week. Which ones are unproductive (focused on the distant future, beyond your control to solve, unlikely to occur) and which are productive (focused on the near future, within your control to solve, likely to occur)? Write a *U* next to each unproductive worry and a *P* next to each productive one. Remember that you'll probably find both types of worries recorded in your worry diary.

Step Three: Change Your Thinking

In chapter 5, you learned that your thoughts largely determine how you feel. You also learned that, when you have negative feelings, such as anxiety, your thoughts are often distorted in some way. Though worries can contain many thought distortions, three are particularly common:

- **Fortune telling.** This is the essence of worry. You are predicting the future. For instance, when Olivia quit her job to raise her newborn twins, she felt intense anxiety. She told herself things like "We won't be able to afford college" and "We'll have to move back in with my parents." These thoughts are good examples of fortune telling.

- **Catastrophic thinking.** This is the catastrophic component of worry. You exaggerate how awful the thing you fear would be if it came true. For example, Claire, a mother of a six-month-old boy, was told she'd have to travel for work more. She felt extremely anxious because she thought, "I'll never see him again. He's going to grow up without a mom."

- **Discounting your coping skills.** You create anxiety by underestimating your ability to cope with problems. You tell yourself harmful things such as "I can't handle it" or "I can't stand it; it's too much."

How to Change Your Worry Thoughts

Once you've decided that a particular worry is unproductive and distorted in some way, you'll need to challenge it and change the way you think about it. Remember that cognitive therapy is based on the idea that our thoughts influence our feelings. To change how you feel, you must change how you think.

In chapter 5, we listed several general techniques that you can use to change your thinking and lessen your anxiety. In this section, we'll show you how to apply these cognitive techniques to worry and use them to defeat your fears. Let's begin by looking at the first one, countering catastrophic thinking, and then we'll look at three more ways to turn your thinking around.

1. **Counter catastrophic thinking.** One antidote to worry is to ask yourself a series of questions designed to "decatastrophize" your thinking. To give this technique a try, first take out a sheet of paper. At the top, write down the worry that's troubling you. Then, below, answer the following questions about this worry:

   - What is the worst-case scenario?

   - How likely is it that the worst-case scenario will come true?

   - What could I do to cope if the worst-case scenario did occur?

   - What are at least three other possible outcomes?

   - What is the most likely outcome?

   - How often have I been right in the past when I've predicted disaster?

Here's how Samantha used this technique to deflate one of her worries:

Countering Catastrophic Thinking
Worry: Once I have a baby and go on maternity leave, my career will be over.

What is the worst-case scenario? I end up permanently unemployed, we have to cut our expenses way back, we burn through our savings, and our daughter has to take out loans for college.

How likely is it that the worst-case scenario will come true? Not very likely. I'll find some kind of work.

What could I do to cope if the worst-case scenario did occur? I could make the best of it. We can still have a lot of fun and build a great family without a lot of money.

What are at least three other possible outcomes?

- I stay at the same job, but I don't get promoted as fast.
- I leave this job to find another that better fits my goals and values.
- I start my own business.

What is the most likely outcome? I stay at this job and strive for a balance between my work and my home life.

How often have I been right in the past when I've predicted disaster? Never.

2. **Examine the evidence.** When we worry, we often treat our negative thoughts as if they are true without considering the facts. Examining the evidence encourages healthy skepticism about your thinking. The following questions can help you test out your worry thoughts. Give them a try: put your own thoughts to the test and see if they are really true:

- What specific event am I predicting?
- What is the evidence that supports this prediction?
- What is the evidence that does not support this prediction?
- Which side is more convincing?
- What should I do now?

Samantha also used this technique to counter her fear that she'd lose her job after having a baby. Here's how she did it:

Examining the Evidence

Worry: Once I have a baby and go on maternity leave, my career will be over.

What specific event am I predicting? I'll get fired after I return from maternity leave.

What is the evidence that supports this prediction? One of my friends at another company didn't seem to get promoted as quickly after having a child.

What is the evidence that does not support this prediction?

- To my knowledge, no one has gotten fired for taking maternity leave in our company.

- Several of my colleagues have had children, taken maternity leave, and returned to their careers without any significant effects.

- I discussed this with my boss and she assured me that it wouldn't hurt my career.

- My boss has three children of her own.

- Our company strives to be supportive of families and working mothers.

- Discriminating against a woman for taking maternity leave is illegal.

Which side is more convincing? The evidence against.

What should I do now? Have my baby, take my maternity leave, and enjoy this special time. Then I can return to work and strive for a good work-life balance.

---

3. **Do a cost-benefit analysis.** Sometimes overcoming worry comes down to making a choice: is it better to (1) suffer from the chronic, nagging pain of worrying, or (2) just deal with the emotional pain later in the unlikely event that your worst fear comes true? In the end, does worrying about uncontrollable possible future events really do any good anyway?

One way to find out is to do a cost-benefit analysis. To do a cost-benefit analysis, simply take out a sheet of paper and draw a line down the middle. On the left column, write "Costs" and on the right column, write "Benefits." Then list all the costs and benefits of worrying about a particular issue on your sheet. Once you've done this, take a minute to analyze them. Which side wins? Is it more to your benefit or detriment to worry?

For example, one day Rachel took her four-month-old son, Johnny, to a carnival. While on a ride, they sat next to another mom with a son who was about Johnny's age. The woman told Rachel that her son had a rare and fatal disease and she was taking him out one last time. It was a sad ride; Rachel held back tears for much of it. In the weeks that followed, the image of the mother and her son haunted Rachel. She found herself worrying, "What if that happens to Johnny? What if he gets some terrible disease? I couldn't live with that. I couldn't handle it." Rachel decided to use a cost-benefit analysis to see if the costs of worrying outweighed its benefits. Here's what she came up with:

Cost-Benefit Analysis	
Worry: My son will die of a rare disease.	
Costs	**Benefits**
1. I'm ruining the present with my worry about the future. 2. I feel tense and anxious. 3. I have trouble sleeping. 4. I feel irritable and stressed. 5. I'm wasting energy on worrying. 6. I'm running to the doctor for everything. 7. I'm spending large chunks of time researching diseases and symptoms on the Internet. 8. I'm teaching my son to worry.	1. I'm more vigilant for signs of disease so I'll act faster if something happens. 2. I could catch it early if he were to get sick. 3. I show how much I love my son by worrying so much about him.

After looking at her list, two things became clear to Rachel. The first was that her worry actually had some benefits. Prior to doing this analysis, all Rachel knew was that her worry was uncomfortable and she wanted it to stop. Like Rachel, many people are surprised to learn that problems such as worry often have an upside.

Even with the benefits she identified, Rachel saw—for the first time—just how much her worry was costing her. She was able to step back and see that she was paying a huge price in the form of lack of joy, lost sleep, and irritability. But for Rachel to give up her worry, she'd have to take a risk. She'd have to give up some of her worry and vigilance about her son's health. The benefits of giving up her worry might include relaxing and enjoying her child, and building a life-long bond based on love and joy not overprotection and worry. She'd be able to respond more effectively to her child's needs, connect more deeply with him, and provide a calm, relaxed role model. The tradeoff is that she *might* react less quickly to signs of an illness than she would have if she worried and checked constantly.

You'll face a similar decision if your cost-benefit analysis reveals that your worry is more harmful than helpful. If you choose to give up your worry, you might have to expose yourself to more risk. Only you can decide if it's worth it. Ask yourself whether the drawbacks of worrying about something bad happening outweigh the benefits of constantly being on guard. Doing a cost-benefit analysis can help you make an informed decision.

It's important to note that, even if your cost-benefit analysis shows that your worry and anxiety is clearly working against you, this doesn't mean your worry will evaporate. For instance, Rachel might still feel anxious from time to time when she decides not to scrutinize her son's health. But your cost-benefit analysis—one that shows all the ways worry and anxiety harm you and your child—can give you the strength to fight your fears and defeat them.

4. Double standard. Another technique you can use to turn your worry around is called the "double standard." As we discussed in chapter 5, the essence of this technique is to give yourself the same advice you would offer a close friend. Remember that we're often much more objective and helpful to others than we are to ourselves.

To try the double standard technique, take out a sheet of paper and draw a line down the middle. On the left side, record your worries. Now take a look at those worries and imagine that a close friend came to you with those same fears, asking you for advice. What would you tell her? How would you comfort her and make her feel better? Remember, this is a good friend, so you want to be honest with her. You want to tell her the truth but also help her and make her feel comfortable.

Here's how Kristen used the double standard technique to calm her fears about having a child:

| Double Standard Technique ||
Worry	What Would I Tell a Close Friend?
I've never been a mom before. How will I know what to do? My mom was not a good example. I'll probably screw my baby up permanently. I can't even change a diaper. This is going to be a disaster.	You'll learn on the job. You can do it. You might make some mistakes, but everyone does. You love your child and that's the most important thing. Plus, if you have any trouble, you can ask your husband or friends for help.

Once you've filled in the right side of the column, ask yourself, "Is this good advice?" "Do I agree with it and believe it?" If you answer yes, can you apply the same caring, helpful advice to yourself?

Exercise: Change Your Thinking

Choose an unproductive worry from your worry diary and use the four techniques described above, in How to Change Your Worry Thoughts, to challenge and change your thinking. Be sure to try them all. You might have to try two, three, or all four before you turn your worry around and change the way you feel. You can also refer to chapter 5 for additional strategies.

Step Four: Practice Exposure and Response Prevention

As you learned in chapter 6, exposure and response prevention (ERP) is a highly effective way to overcome some anxiety problems. Exposure means directly confronting the thing you fear; response prevention means eliminating any behaviors that reduce your anxiety. In this step, you'll learn how to apply these two techniques to worry.

Using Exposure to Conquer Worry

Direct exposure is one of the best ways to overcome something that you fear. However, at times direct exposure is neither desirable nor practical. For example, let's suppose you are worried that you and your baby will die in a car accident. Confronting this worry by making an accident happen would hardly be a smart way to overcome it!

There is a way, however, to practice exposure with worries when using direct exposure won't work: imaginal exposure. As you'll recall from reading chapter 6, imaginal exposure means facing your worst fear in your imagination, not in real life. Although you might not think that using your imagination to confront your fears would be strong enough medicine to allow you to overcome them, you might be in for a surprise. Imaginal exposure can be a remarkably powerful technique.

To use imaginal exposure to defeat an unproductive worry, write a narrative script describing your worst fear coming true. Your script should be a first-person account of about one to three pages that includes as much detail as possible, such as sights, sounds, smells, textures, and emotions.

When creating your script, try to follow these two rules:

1. It has to be the absolute worst-case scenario. Don't hold back. Bring out your inner Stephen King and try to make your script as frightening as possible.

2. The rules of logic don't apply. Even if your worst fear doesn't make logical sense, write it down anyway. Your goal is to capture your worst fear on paper in vivid detail.

Once you've created your script, practice reading it for about twenty to thirty minutes each day. Or, if you prefer, you can record yourself reading your script out loud and listen to it if this makes it easier for you to focus on visualizing your story. Continue practicing until you can read or listen to your script and vividly imagine your worst fear coming true with little or no anxiety.

Meg used this technique to overcome her worry that her daughter, Sophia, would die of pneumonia. Meg confronted this fear by creating an imaginal script, with Sophia contracting pneumonia, getting sick, going to the hospital, and ultimately succumbing to the disease. Her script was quite graphic and included vivid descriptions of upsetting images that were difficult even for her therapist to read!

Even though Meg's script laid out her worst fears in exact detail and caused her tremendous anxiety at first, she repeatedly practiced reading it and imagining her worst-case scenario coming true. After much practice, Meg was able to imagine her worst-case scenario with no anxiety. Meg also noticed that she worried much less as a result.

Exercise: Practice Imaginal Exposure

Create a script that describes your worst fear coming true. Then practice imagining your worst-case scenario for twenty to thirty minutes each day. Keep at it until you can read your script without feeling anxiety.

How to Use Response Prevention to Defeat Your Worry

As we discussed earlier, worry consists of catastrophic thoughts about the future. There is, however, another element of worry that we haven't mentioned much yet: it's what you do *after* you worry. As we noted in chapter 3, worry often leads to what are known as *worry behaviors* —any action that you take in response to your worry. One study found that about half of all worries lead to some sort of worry behavior (Craske et al. 1989). Worry behaviors make you feel better by temporarily lessening your anxiety; however, they maintain your worry in the long run, making you miserable in the process.

You may recognize some of the following common worry behaviors from chapter 6:

- **Reassurance seeking.** This is one of the most common worry behaviors, often consisting of asking for reassurance from friends, family members, doctors, or other people you trust. You might also seek reassurance from parenting books or websites.

- **Checking.** As the name suggests, this type of worry behavior involves repeatedly checking in response to worry. For instance, if you're pregnant you might purchase a home heartbeat monitor so you can check your baby's heartbeat whenever you feel anxious.

- **Superstitions.** These worry behaviors are attempts to prevent your fears from coming true, but they usually have no direct connection to your worry. For example, one mom always put her daughter's socks on right foot first because she felt that putting them on left foot first would bring bad luck. Another mom would only give her son an even number of spoonfuls of cereal because she felt odd numbers would cause something bad to happen. By performing these actions, you convince yourself that you've decreased or eliminated risk. Practically speaking, however, these behaviors have no real impact on the likelihood of your worry coming true.

- **Overprotection.** If you're worried about your baby's health or safety, you might go to extremes to protect him, perhaps shielding him from all direct sunlight or preventing other people from ever holding him.

- **Avoidance.** Some people respond to their worry by simply avoiding everything associated with that worry. For example, you might switch to another channel when a news story about pregnancy risks comes on, or you might change the subject when another mom starts talking about something that makes you anxious.

Exercise: Identify and Eliminate Your Worry Behaviors

Now that you are familiar with worry behaviors, follow these two steps to rid yourself of these problematic behaviors:

1. **Identify your worry behaviors.** Using the list below, make a check mark next to any behaviors you've used to cope with your worry:

   ☐ Reassurance seeking ☐ Superstitions

   ☐ Checking ☐ Avoidance

   ☐ Overprotection

2. **Eliminate your worry behaviors.** Now that you've identified your worry behaviors, it's time to eliminate them. The next time worry strikes, you'll feel a powerful urge to resort to these old, ineffective ways of managing worry. To truly get control over your worry, be stubborn and resist these behaviors. You'll feel your anxiety rise and tempt you to give in. Hang in there! Your anxiety—and worry—will eventually fade away, and you'll experience peace of mind and a renewed sense of control over your worry.

Note: To stop using avoidance and superstition you'll need to use a variation on this technique. If you rely on avoidance, you'll want to expose yourself to the source of your worry. And if you are using superstitious behaviors, you'll want to do the opposite of the superstition. For example, if you feel that dressing your child in a black shirt would mean "bad luck," you'll want to practice dressing your child in a black shirt until it no longer causes anxiety.

In the short term, eliminating these behaviors might cause you to feel more anxiety. But in the long run, you'll feel much less anxious. If you're unsure about resisting these worry behaviors, ask yourself this: have they put an end to your worry, or are they just a temporary fix? If your worry behaviors only work in the short run, give response prevention a try. It could be the technique that helps you conquer your worry once and for all.

> ~ COMMON QUESTION ~
> **What can I do instead of engaging in worry behaviors?**
>
> When you are eliminating a worry behavior, it can be helpful to replace it with something new. So what can you do instead of engaging in these worry behaviors? Try something that relaxes you, such as the calming activities and techniques mentioned earlier in this chapter. These activities are an excellent replacement for worry behaviors.

Step Five: Accept Uncertainty

Ever wonder how some moms cruise through pregnancy and postpartum without a care, while others are wracked with worry? The answer may lie in the ability to tolerate *uncertainty*. According to some exciting research, those who can deal with uncertainty worry less than those who are intolerant of the unknown and need guarantees in life (Ladouceur, Gosselin, and Dugas 2000).

For example, Holly's daughter, Charlotte, was born a few weeks premature. Though Charlotte was healthy, she was tiny at birth, weighing just over four pounds. To Holly, Charlotte looked so small and frail as she slept in the hospital nursery. Soon after Holly brought Charlotte home from the hospital, her protective maternal instincts kicked in and she found herself worrying constantly that Charlotte would die. She worried about illnesses, falls, car accidents, food allergies, choking, and electrical outlets. In the first few months of Charlotte's life, Holly felt that she had imagined almost every possible catastrophe that could befall her daughter.

Eventually, however, Holly came to accept that she just couldn't predict the future. Would Charlotte live to age ten? Fifty? One hundred? Holly admitted that she didn't know, and no one else knew either. She finally had to accept the uncertainty that comes with a child. She became determined to enjoy every minute with Charlotte and not let her worry spoil her experience of motherhood. Holly even started telling herself, "If she dies, I'll just have to deal with it then. I'm going to enjoy the present instead of worrying."

Holly's response might seem callous and uncaring, but it was actually a healthy reaction. By accepting the uncertainty, Holly was able to relax and enjoy the time she had with her child. It also freed her up to be a better parent. None of us knows just how much time we'll get with our children. By accepting some uncertainty about the future, you can free yourself to live each moment to the fullest.

Exercise: Accept Uncertainty

The next time you notice a "what if" thought popping up in your head, refuse to answer it. Counter it instead with responses that acknowledge rather than squash uncertainty, such as the following:

- "Maybe it will; maybe it won't."

- "I'll never know for sure."

- "I can't predict the future."

- "Anything is possible."

- "Nothing ventured, nothing gained."

- Risk is a part of life.

Next Steps

Once you've tried all five steps we listed in this chapter, take a moment to assess how you feel. If you've restored some peace to your life and you feel your worry is under control, congratulations! You've worked hard and earned the spoils of victory. If you're still feeling more anxious than you would like, consider going back through the steps again and giving it another try.

Or, if your anxiety is partially based on one of the other problems in this book, like panic or post-traumatic stress, you can go to the chapters related to those problems and apply the techniques we've described there as well. Remember, persistence and hard work are the keys. Keep at it until your anxiety is under control.

Key Points

- Worry is defined as catastrophic thinking about the future. Excessive and chronic worry can cause physical, emotional, and relationship problems.

- New and expectant moms typically worry about four key things: labor and delivery, the health of their child, the impact of a child on their life, and their competence as a mother.

- There are five key steps to the process of conquering worry: practicing relaxation, determining whether your worry is productive, challenging unproductive worries, practicing exposure and response prevention, and accepting uncertainty.

- By applying these five steps, you can overcome your tendency to worry and restore peace and joy to your life.

CHAPTER 11

Deal with Trauma

Delivering a child is one of the most beautiful, wondrous things imaginable. It's also one of the hardest and most frightening. For some women, the process of labor and delivery can be traumatizing in and of itself. In other cases, anxiety or fear stemming from past traumas like childhood sexual abuse, rape, or assault can be triggered by pregnancy and delivery.

In this chapter, you'll learn how to identify symptoms of post-traumatic stress, apply relaxation skills when facing anxiety triggers, challenge distorted beliefs, and change patterns of behavior that maintain your fear. You cannot change what has happened in the past, nor can you avoid labor and delivery, but you *can* learn to cope better and decrease your fear and avoidance. Your step-by-step plan for dealing with trauma will reduce your anxiety symptoms by helping you confront your fears and change your reactions to stressful events.

What Is Post-traumatic Stress?

Although post-traumatic stress is often associated with men who have served in war, post-traumatic stress is actually much more common and more chronic in women than it is in men. Rape, childhood sexual abuse, domestic violence, and labor and delivery are some of the experiences that can cause a post-traumatic stress reaction in women, but this type of reaction can occur whenever a person feels terrified and helpless in a situation. As we discussed in chapter 3, primary symptoms of post-traumatic stress include reexperiencing the event, avoidance and numbing, and increased arousal (American Psychiatric Association 2000).

Reexperiencing the trauma can occur through any the following:

- Intrusive thoughts, images, or ideas about the trauma

- Nightmares or bad dreams about or related to the event

- Flashbacks—acting or feeling like it is happening again

- Extreme physical or emotional reactions when reminded of the trauma

Avoidance or numbing can include the following:

- Avoiding people, situations, or activities that remind you of the traumatic event

- Not thinking or talking about the trauma

- Avoiding feelings associated with the trauma

- Feeling emotionally numb or unable to experience emotions

- Isolating yourself from important activities and people

- Loss of memory of major parts of the traumatic event

Symptoms of increased arousal may include the following:

- Problems falling or staying asleep

- Excessive irritability or outbursts of anger

- Trouble concentrating

- Hypervigilance, or extreme alertness, to your environment

- Exaggerated startle response—feeling jumpy, edgy, or easily startled

Not everyone who goes through a trauma will have post-traumatic stress, and it is normal to temporarily experience some of these symptoms in response to a highly stressful event. However, if these symptoms interfere with your life or when they do not resolve on their own, you may be experiencing post-traumatic stress disorder (PTSD). PTSD can begin within several weeks of the trauma, or it may not appear until months or even years later.

PTSD in Pregnancy and the Postpartum Period

Around 10 percent of women will receive a diagnosis of PTSD in their lifetime (Kessler et al. 1995). Studies have found that, during pregnancy, around 3 percent of women meet diagnostic criteria for PTSD (Rogal et al. 2007; Smith et al. 2006), and for women at six weeks postpartum PTSD estimates vary from 2.8 to 5.6 percent (Ayers and Pickering 2001; Creedy, Schochet, and Horsfall 2000). PTSD during pregnancy is a serious concern because it can be associated with substance use, preterm delivery, and other psychological problems, such as depression (Rogal et al. 2007).

Women can have symptoms of post-traumatic stress as a result of events unrelated to pregnancy, such as childhood abuse, domestic violence, rape, or assault. Or, their symptoms may result from a pregnancy-related trauma such as stillbirth, miscarriage, or premature birth. In fact, even a full-term pregnancy with a healthy outcome can lead to post-traumatic stress in some cases.

Many women perceive childbirth as traumatic, even when labor occurs in a normal fashion and the delivery is healthy. Women may have intense feelings of being out of control of the situation or they may fear that the baby might be harmed in the process. In addition, labor pain can be traumatizing for some women, particularly if pain relief strategies are ineffective. And very long deliveries or those with complications can cause distress or intense anxiety, especially when accompanied by a lack of information or support from obstetric staff or family. Finally, women may have expectations about childbirth that are not met, or they may have had previous traumatic delivery experiences. Any of these factors can lead to the development of a post-traumatic stress reaction following the birth of a child.

Recognizing Post-Traumatic Stress after Delivery

Keep in mind that it is common to experience some of these symptoms after a stressful event like childbirth and they usually resolve on their own after some time. However, if you have many of the symptoms listed above, they interfere in your life, and they do not appear to be going away, you may consider them a post-traumatic stress reaction or even full-blown PTSD. If you continue to have nightmares about or intrusive memories of labor and delivery, feel emotionally detached from or avoid contact with your baby, avoid reading or talking about childbirth, or worry excessively about getting pregnant again, you may find the strategies outlined in this chapter helpful.

~ COMMON QUESTION ~

What might put me at risk for PTSD?

A number of risk factors have been identified in the development of PTSD and PTSD-like symptoms following childbirth, including:

- History of psychological problems
- Tendency to be anxious
- Difficult delivery
- Negative contact with medical staff during labor and delivery
- Feelings of loss of control
- Lack of partner support

Identify and Track Your Symptoms

If you have been the victim of a trauma, you may find that you have some of the symptoms discussed above. Put a check mark in the box next to any of the following symptoms of post-traumatic stress that you are currently experiencing:

☐ Intrusive thoughts, images, or ideas about the trauma

☐ Nightmares or bad dreams about and/or related to the event

☐ Flashbacks—acting or feeling like it is happening again

☐ Extreme physical or emotional reactions when reminded of the trauma

☐ Avoiding situations, activities, or people that remind you of the event

☐ Not thinking or talking about the event

☐ Avoid feelings associated with the trauma

☐ Feeling emotionally numb or unable to experience emotions

☐ Isolating yourself from important activities and people

☐ Loss of memory for major parts of the traumatic event

☐ Problems falling or staying asleep

☐ Excessive irritability or anger outbursts

☐ Trouble concentrating

☐ Hypervigilance, or extreme alertness, to your environment

☐ Exaggerated startle response—feeling jumpy or edgy, or feeling startled easily

Do you have a lot of these symptoms? If so, the steps outlined below may be helpful to you. If you also experience other symptoms like depression, if you use alcohol or drugs to cope with your anxiety, or if you have thoughts of harming yourself, talk to your obstetrician, therapist, or other trusted care provider right away.

Exercise: Track Your Symptoms

For the next week, keep track of your post-traumatic stress symptoms using the form on the next page. Make as many photocopies as you need to record the date, time, and situation in which your symptoms occur. Write down any triggers that you notice, and rate the intensity of your anxiety. Check off your avoidance behaviors and be sure to write down your thoughts in each situation.

Look back at your records over the past week, and ask yourself the questions below:

Did you notice any triggers for your anxiety? _____

_____

Were your symptoms more likely to occur in certain situations?_____

_____

Was any physical sensation or thought more likely to initiate your anxiety?_____

_____

What were your most troubling or most frequent symptoms?_____

_____

Did you escape from or avoid any situations? If so, which ones?_____

_____

Symptom Monitoring Form

Date and Time: _____

Situation/Trigger: _____

Anxiety   **Level**
(circle)

0	10	20	30	40	50	60	70	80	90	100

Not Anxious   **Moderately Anxious**   **Very Anxious**

☐ Nightmares or bad dreams   ☐ Strong emotional reaction

☐ Trouble concentrating   ☐ Feeling numb

☐ Intrusive thoughts or images   ☐ Strong physical reaction

☐ Hypervigilance to surroundings   ☐ Irritability or anger

☐ Flashbacks   ☐ Problems sleeping

☐ Jumpy, edgy, startled easily

What I thought: _____

_____

_____

What I avoided:

Situations or activities that I associate with the event

People who remind me of the trauma

Thinking about the event

Talking about the event

Feelings that I associate with the event

People or activities that are important to me

Other:_____

Other:_____

Your Five-Step Plan to Cope with Post-traumatic Stress

Now that you have identified any symptoms of PTSD you may have and have monitored them for at least one week, you're ready to use the skills you learned in part 2 of this book to begin to change your reactions. In this section, we'll describe five key steps to coping with post-traumatic stress during and after pregnancy:

1. Communicate with your obstetrician.

2. Use your relaxation skills.

3. Challenge any distorted thoughts.

4. Confront feared memories.

5. Face avoided situations.

Step One: Communicate with Your Obstetrician

The first step in ensuring a pregnancy, delivery, and postpartum period that are free from the effects of post-traumatic stress is to talk with your obstetrician. If you are pregnant and have any of the risk factors we described above, don't delay. Although it may be difficult, speaking openly with your doctor will benefit both you and your unborn child. Your medical provider can help you in the areas listed below by doing the following:

- **Assisting you in preparing for labor and delivery.** It's good to be prepared, but labor and delivery rarely go exactly as planned. Your medical provider can help you prepare in a realistic way, so you can have a general idea of what to expect but are ready to be flexible. Resist making overly detailed plans that may add to your anxiety if things don't go as expected.

- **Informing you ahead of time about possible complications or procedures.** It may be helpful to be familiar with procedures that may arise during labor and delivery. However, remember that not every possibility can be anticipated in advance.

- **Ensuring that obstetric staff communicate clearly with you.** Your medical practitioner may be able to ask staff to talk directly with you and let you know what's going on. However, you may also be an advocate for yourself by making direct, specific requests of the staff, like "Please explain to me what is happening now," or "I'd like you to let me know before you touch me."

- **Discussing your pain management plan well in advance of your due date.** Be sure to discuss your options and have a backup plan in place in the event that, when the time comes, your preferred choice is not possible.

- **Making sure you have an adequate social support plan for labor and delivery.** Be sure you have someone to help guide you through the labor and delivery process. Ideally, this person should be aware of any trauma history you have so they can also act as a liaison between you and medical staff if need be.

- **Referring you to an appropriate mental health provider for treatment, if necessary.** If you have a history of sexual abuse or assault, or if you feel for any reason that you could have a traumatic reaction to childbirth, you may find it helpful to work with a therapist to prepare for labor and delivery. Ask your obstetrician for referrals or look at the list of resources at the end of this book for options.

Being proactive is the best strategy for preventing an adverse reaction following the birth of your child. It can give your baby the best start possible and help you enter motherhood with maximum joy and minimum trauma.

If you've already delivered your baby and are struggling with post-traumatic stress symptoms, a discussion with your obstetrician or another trusted healthcare provider will still be beneficial. The physical sensations of childbirth and breastfeeding can sometimes trigger trauma-related memories and uncomfortable feelings or emotions. Your obstetrician can point you toward support groups or other resources that may help you heal.

Exercise: Talk to Your Doctor

Schedule an appointment to meet with your doctor. Be sure to let the receptionist know that you may need a longer block of time for this discussion; you might ask for the first or last appointment of the day if that would allow you more time with the doctor. Before you go, make notes regarding any important points you want to tell your doctor about or any questions you may have. Take a support person along with you, if you'd like. It may be hard for you to have this conversation, but know that you are doing what's best for you and for your baby.

Step Two: Use Your Relaxation Skills

The second step in coping with symptoms of post-traumatic stress is to work on your relaxation skills. In chapter 4, you learned relaxation strategies to address the physical sensations of anxiety, and you may find any of these techniques to be useful. However, we find that our clients who suffer symptoms of PTSD seem to benefit most from using either diaphragmatic breathing or progressive muscle relaxation to deal with their anxiety.

Look back at chapter 4 and review the instructions for diaphragmatic breathing and progressive muscle relaxation. Continue to practice these techniques each day until you feel comfortable with them. You will then be ready to use these skills to both address any physical sensations that trigger your symptoms and cope with your anxiety.

Step Three: Challenge Distorted Thoughts

In chapter 5, you discovered how powerful our thoughts can be in influencing our emotions. If you have gone through a trauma, this experience can have a particularly strong impact on your thoughts—how you view yourself, the world, and the future. You may have thoughts about the world being dangerous, events being out of your control, or life being extremely fragile. These thoughts can in turn have a powerful effect on how you feel, leading to anxiety, avoidance, and fear. Below, we review a few common thought distortions that can lead to anxiety but you may also go back and look at the entire list in chapter 5.

All-or-Nothing Thinking

You see the world in extreme, black-or-white categories, such as "good or bad" or "perfect or a failure." Sondra, a victim of childhood sexual abuse, was now six months pregnant with her first child. Though she wanted to receive good care for her baby, she believed that "no man can be trusted." As a result, she avoided checkups with her obstetrician because some of the nurses in the office were male.

Overgeneralization

You make broad inferences based on just one or a few events. Laura is pregnant with her second child and choosing a hospital for her delivery. During her first delivery, she had a negative interaction with one of the staff members. For this second delivery, she refuses to return to that hospital, even though it is close to her home and has an excellent reputation, because she thinks "the staff there are all jerks."

Overestimating the Threat

You take a situation that involves slight or no risk and make it seem threatening and dangerous. Joanna grew up in a tough neighborhood, where she witnessed harm coming to many friends and family members. Although she now lives in a very safe area with a low crime rate, she won't take her new baby for walks in the stroller because she believes "it is not safe."

Catastrophic Thinking

You take a minor setback and view it as horrible, awful, or terrible. Mona had a detailed plan for how her labor and delivery would go. When the doctor informed her that a C-section would be necessary, she was devastated, thinking, "This is terrible way to enter motherhood."

Discounting Your Coping Skills

You tell yourself that you can't cope with problems or difficulties. During the birth of her first child, Sarah's pain control was ineffective; however, she managed to get through labor and delivered a healthy child. However, now pregnant with her second, she is anxious and fearful, thinking, "I can't possibly do that again."

"Should" Statements

You set rigid, absolute rules for yourself and others about how things "should" and "shouldn't" be. Larissa, who had high expectations for herself, had a long and difficult delivery and afterward felt guilty, disappointed, and angry with herself, because she thought, "I should've been able to manage my delivery better."

Look closely at the thoughts you have written down on your symptom monitoring forms, above. Do you see any of these distortions in your thoughts?

Changing Your Thoughts

Now it's time to challenge those distortions and lower your anxiety. In chapter 5, we described several techniques for changing your thinking, and you can use any of them to counter your anxious thoughts. Remember Sondra, who was sexually abused as a child and was now pregnant and having difficulty trusting male health care providers? Below is one of Sondra's Cognitive Therapy Worksheets showing how she coped with her distorted thoughts related to her past trauma.

Upsetting Event	Feelings	Anxious Thoughts	Cognitive Distortions	Coping Responses
Upcoming appointment for my 6-month OB checkup	Anxious Angry	Just my luck—I'll probably get that male nurse when it's time to take my blood pressure.	Fortune telling	There are many female nurses on staff, so it is more likely that I will get a female. I can always request to work with a female if I want to.
		I can't trust men.	All-or-nothing thinking	I know several men I can trust. The fact that one man was not trustworthy doesn't mean they all are bad.
		I am in danger.	Overestimating the threat	The doctor's office is a professional place with lots of people around. I'll be safe there.

As you'll recall, Sarah was a mom who was traumatized by the difficult delivery of her first child. She now is anxious and doubtful of her ability to manage that process again. On the next page is Sarah's thought record:

Upsetting Event	Feelings	Anxious Thoughts	Cognitive Distortions	Coping Responses
Talking with my husband about our due date	Anxious Fearful	My last delivery was terrible.	Catastrophic thinking, all-or-nothing thinking	My last delivery was really hard, but there were some moments that were exciting too, and it was definitely worth it.
		No way can I do that again.	Fortune telling, discounting my coping skills	It is scary, but I was scared last time too. I managed to get through it before and I have a beautiful baby to show for it.
		What if it is too painful and I can't stand it?	Catastrophic thinking, discounting my coping skills	Childbirth can be painful but I have gotten through it before. I can talk to my OB ahead of time and choose different pain relief options that might make a difference.

Now it's your turn. Make copies of the form on the next page or record the information in a notebook or journal. Pick a recent thought from your recording forms and use the strategies in chapter 5 to help you generate coping responses.

Exercise: Challenge Your Anxious Thoughts

After you have practiced identifying the distortions in one of your previous thoughts and generating coping responses to that thought, you can continue practicing with other past thoughts. Or you may now try to use this method to cope with thoughts as they arise. It will likely be difficult at first, but it will get easier if you stick with it. Practice challenging your thoughts at least once every day.

Step Four: Confront Your Feared Memories

In chapter 6, we discussed exposure therapy and how it can be useful in tackling anxiety problems. Studies have found that this can be a highly effective strategy for dealing with trauma (Foa et al. 1991; Taylor et al. 2003). If you are like most women, though, it probably sounds pretty frightening. Let's take a moment to review the rationale for confronting feared thoughts, or, in the case of traumatic experiences, feared memories.

Upsetting Event	Feelings	Anxious Thoughts	Cognitive Distortions	Coping Responses

Rationale for Exposure to Feared Memories

If you are experiencing symptoms of post-traumatic stress, then by definition you are already thinking about the trauma. The experience comes back to you in the form of intrusive thoughts, nightmares, flashbacks, and high anxiety. You attempt to distract yourself from, ignore, and push away the memories. It is natural to want to avoid distressing and upsetting recollections. But how has that worked for you so far? As we discussed in detail in chapter 6, this is a highly ineffective strategy. If it worked well, you wouldn't be experiencing nightmares or having intrusive thoughts of the trauma. Symptoms of post-traumatic stress thrive on avoidance and fear. In order to correctly process and file away these memories for good, you must first confront them. When you confront your memories of the trauma, the anxiety you feel in response to them will gradually decrease or habituate. You will soon learn that you can tolerate thinking about or talking about the trauma. It will be difficult at first—sometimes you may even experience more anxiety temporarily—but it will get easier if you keep with it. Eventually you will see anxiety's grip on your life slowly loosen.

Creating Your Imaginal Exposure Script

Sarah addressed her traumatic memories of childbirth using *imaginal exposure*. Remember, imaginal exposure means that you are practicing exposures in your imagination or in your mind. Using the steps below, you can create an imaginal exposure script to conquer your fear, anxiety, and avoidance:

1. Write a detailed script about the trauma. Be as detailed as possible and tell the story in the present tense, as if it is happening right now.

2. Record the story onto an audiotape or digital recorder.

3. Listen to the story repeatedly until your anxiety decreases.

Sarah's imaginal script of her traumatic delivery looked something like this:

It is early on a Monday morning and I arrive at the hospital with my husband after a few hours of mild contractions. Everyone is really nice as we check in on the OB floor, and I am directed to a room where I change into my hospital gown and booties. We settle in and listen to some music as a constant stream of nurses and medical residents come into ask questions and monitor the baby. They tell me I am 5 centimeters dilated and I am surprised that it doesn't hurt more. I decline the epidural for now since I am not really in much pain yet, thinking there will be plenty of time for that later. It is quiet in our room now. My husband and I work on a crossword, joking and excited about meeting our new baby. After a half an hour or so, though, things start to get bad. The contractions are coming faster now and they hurt a lot more. I call for the nurse and it seems like it takes forever for her to get there. When she arrives, I ask her to get the anesthesiologist and get me that epidural right away. She promises to call, but it seems like I'm waiting forever. Finally, my OB comes. She takes a look and says that I am fully dilated and that I need to start pushing. She says that the anesthesiologist has been called to a surgery and there is no time anyway, that we need to get the baby out. I am crying now and I'm so scared. My doctor and the nurses rush around the room and I am terrified that something is wrong with my baby. I ask and ask but no one is answering me; they are so focused on the baby. I can barely stand the pain and I am screaming for my husband to do something to make this stop. He looks pale and shaken and I think for sure that something is terribly wrong. I feel so helpless and out of control. I never imagined that it could hurt this much. Everything is a blur. I feel like this will never end.

After writing out this recollection of her delivery, Sarah recorded it onto an audiotape and listened to it each day. She used the form below to record her anxiety as she listened to it. In each of her exposure sessions, she repeatedly listened to the story while remembering it as vividly as possible. This was extremely difficult for her initially. She reported her anxiety as a ninety-five and was tearful and distressed as she listened to this memory. With time and repeated exposure, though, her anxiety decreased. She began to more easily tolerate remembering and, as a result, she found that she thought about the delivery less and less. Her nightmares became less frequent, and she was able to talk with her husband about the new baby's arrival without feeling as anxious.

Exercise: Use Imaginal Exposure to Confront Feared Memories

Write a detailed script of your traumatic event and record it on a tape or digital recorder. Listen to the story repeatedly and imagine it as vividly as possible until your anxiety decreases. Use the exposure form below to rate your anxiety and keep track of your progress. In each exposure session, remember to keep listening until your anxiety goes down by about half of its starting point on that day. Try to do sessions on most days, until you can listen to the story with little or no distress.

Exposure Practice Form

Date: _____

Start time: _____   End time: _____

Anxiety level (0 to 100):

Start: _____   Notes: _____

10 minutes: _____   _____

20 minutes: _____   _____

30 minutes: _____   _____

40 minutes: _____   _____

50 minutes: _____   _____

60 minutes: _____   _____

End: _____   _____

Step Five: Face Situations You Avoid

When people experience traumatic events, their behavior often changes to accommodate their new fears. For example, you may avoid situations that are similar to the trauma, that remind you of the trauma, or that are only loosely related to the trauma. In doing so, though, you deprive yourself of the chance to learn that not only can you cope with these situations but your fearful predictions are just not true. In this step, using the strategies discussed in chapter 6, you will learn how to apply exposure therapy to confront the trauma-related situations that you have been avoiding. As you confront these fears, your anxiety will decrease and, over time, you'll notice you can face situations you once avoided with ease.

Your Exposure Hierarchy

Begin by looking at your exposure hierarchy in chapter 6. If you haven't yet created one, use the instructions there to make a list of your feared situations. Put on your list any situations that you avoid, and list your items in order of how much anxiety you would feel if you confronted them, with one hundred being the worst anxiety you can imagine, zero being no anxiety, and fifty indicating moderate anxiety.

Below is an example of Sarah's exposure hierarchy:

Feared Situations	Anxiety
Delivering my baby without an epidural	100
Visiting the hospital OB unit	90
Reading about labor and delivery	85
Going on a tour of the hospital, excluding the OB unit	80
Talking to my husband about our new baby	75
Hearing my friends discuss their childbirth experiences	75
Seeing near-term pregnant women at the grocery store	60
Looking at newborn pictures of my toddler	55
Watching a TV show or movie with a pregnant character	45

After you've completed your hierarchy, select an item that is low on the list—something challenging but not overwhelming. Practice exposing yourself to that situation, and try to stay with it until your anxiety diminishes by about half. This may take twenty minutes or it may take an hour, but it is important that you don't quit before your anxiety comes down. Make copies of the exposure monitoring form from step four so you can use it to rate your anxiety during this exposure exercise. This way you can see your progress over time.

Once an exposure causes you only mild or no anxiety, move up to the next item on your hierarchy and repeat the process until you finish your list. For example, when Sarah started practicing exposure, she rated looking at pictures of her newborn at 55. She looked through photo albums that first day until her anxiety decreased to about 25. Each day that week, she did the same thing until after a few days it no longer caused her much anxiety. She then moved to the next item on her list and continued this way until she had addressed all the items on her hierarchy. If you are having any trouble with the process or your anxiety is not going down, look back at the tips for successful exposures listed near the end of chapter 6.

Exercise: Confront Your Feared Situations

Choose an item low on your hierarchy and begin confronting it daily. Stay with it until your anxiety decreases and then move on to the next item. It will be hard at first, but, with time, your anxiety will decrease. Continue to confront your feared situations until you have completed all items on your list. If you have any questions regarding the safety of confronting the items on your list, be sure to ask your doctor.

Next Steps

After you've tried all five steps we listed in this chapter, take stock of how you are feeling. Has the frequency of your intrusive thoughts or nightmares decreased? Are you less anxious? Do you react differently to situations and things that used to trigger anxiety? Have you stopped avoiding situations that remind you of the trauma? If the answer is yes, good job! You have made important steps toward reclaiming your life. If you're still having trouble, try going back through the steps again or consult a cognitive behavioral therapist in your area. Trauma can be a tough adversary; you may need a good coach on your side to put it in your past once and for all. Ask your obstetrician for help if you have trouble finding a therapist on your own, or refer to list of resources near the end of this book.

Key Points

- Symptoms of post-traumatic stress and full-blown PTSD are common in women and can result from any number of traumatic experiences, including rape, sexual abuse, and domestic violence.

- Even normal labor and delivery with healthy outcomes can lead to PTSD symptoms in some cases.

- If you have a trauma history, working together with your OB to plan your prenatal care and childbirth may minimize adverse effects.

- Challenging any distorted thoughts that may have occurred as a result of the trauma will help to lower your anxiety.

- Directly confronting traumatic memories and avoided situations has been shown to be a very effective treatment for PTSD.

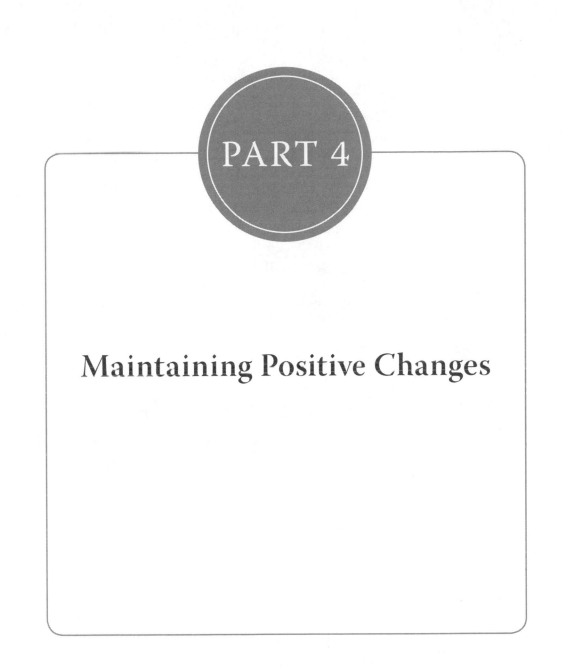

PART 4

Maintaining Positive Changes

CHAPTER 12

Get Support

All people, especially women, have the need to feel connected. Fulfilling relationships with relatives, friends, neighbors, or members of your community are key elements of a meaningful and happy life. At no time are these relationships more important than during your pregnancy and postpartum period. With the sleepless nights, frequent diaper changes, and emotional ups and downs, you'll need some help. Do you have people in your life to whom you can turn for support? We hope your answer is yes! But, if not, don't worry. In this chapter, we'll help you better understand social support, learn why it is so important, and identify ways to get the support and help you need during this important time in your life.

What Is Social Support?

You've probably heard the term "social support," but have you ever really stopped to consider what social support is? It's simple, really. Social support is just someone or something that provides you with emotional or practical assistance. A person—a friend, relative, or spouse—can provide social support, but you can also get social support from groups or from places like church or work. These days, social support doesn't even have to be face-to-face—it can be by e-mail, telephone, or Internet. The options are endless.

Social Support in Pregnancy and the Postpartum Period

Social support is particularly essential during pregnancy and the postpartum period. Having close relationships can improve your health and increase life satisfaction (Balaji et al. 2007) and can even help you to cope more effectively with stress (Glazier et al. 2004). Recent studies have even found that social relationships can protect against postpartum depression (Dennis and Ross 2006), decrease parenting stress (Raikes and Thompson 2005), and improve psychological well-being

(Zachariah 2004). A good social support network can help you to feel better, learn more, and have a healthier relationship with your baby.

Your Five-Step Plan to Good Social Support

Now that you understand how important social support can be to you and your baby, you're ready to use some of the skills you learned in part 2 to learn how to get that support. In this section, we'll describe five steps you can take to improve your support network during pregnancy or the postpartum period. These steps include the following:

1. Understand social support types

2. Evaluate your needs

3. Challenge unsupportive thoughts

4. Ask for the help you need

5. Improve your support network

Step One: Understand Social Support Types

The first step in any search is to decide what you are looking for. There are different kinds of support (Cobb 1976; House 1981): each person in your life will be supportive in his or her own way. Knowing the different types of social support will help you to choose wisely. Here are the different categories of social support:

- **Emotional support.** People who encourage you or support you emotionally are good at listening, make you feel valued, and recognize your strengths.

- **Practical support.** This type of support is one who helps with everyday kinds of problems. These people might assist with babysitting, cooking or cleaning, or finances.

- **Informational support.** This means supports who could offer information, guidance, or advice. They might add input to important decisions you have to make or have special knowledge in a particular area.

- **Peer support.** This type of support is from women who are in the same situation as you or have been through the same experiences. They help by sharing their stories and strategies they've used to get through similar situations.

So, as you can see, different people can be supportive in very different ways. See if you can correctly identify the type of support provided in each of the following examples.

Belinda, a mother of newborn twins, had recently moved to a new city and didn't know many of her neighbors. Her husband worked during the day and she often found it hard to get out of the house. One day, when she was surfing the Internet during her babies' naptime, she found an online chat room for mothers of twins. The "tricks" for parenting twins she found there were particularly helpful to her. She always felt better and less alone after visiting this site and reading the stories posted by other moms.

What type of support did Belinda receive?

☐ Emotional support

☐ Practical support

☐ Informational support

☐ Peer support

~ COMMON QUESTION ~
What if I don't know many people?

The best thing about social support is that a little bit goes a long way. So don't fret if you don't come from a large, close family, if you live in an isolated area, or if you are just plain shy. It doesn't take a lot of social ties to make an impact—it just takes a few good ones. In the next sections, we'll focus on steps you can take to use your existing social supports as well as to develop new ones.

Catherine, seven months pregnant with her first child, was struggling to keep up with her work as a lawyer in a highly competitive firm. Her billable hours had suffered due to the fatigue and nausea she had experienced for much of her pregnancy. She felt like a failure because she was not performing at her previous level. One colleague in particular was very supportive. She often reminded Catherine of how important she was to the firm and how many other women employees had gone through the same temporary professional setbacks during and after pregnancy. At times, she even covered for Catherine at meetings or picked up lunches for them to share. Catherine always felt renewed after talking with this colleague and appreciated her balanced perspective on things.

What type of support did Catherine receive from her colleague?

☐ Emotional support

☐ Practical support

☐ Informational support

☐ Peer support

If you answered that Belinda's online group provided peer support, then you are correct. The online group may also be considered a source of informational support, since she learned parenting skills from the group. What about Catherine's colleague? She certainly provided emotional support, and also some practical support by helping her out at work.

Exercise: Create Your Support Directory

Take out a piece of paper and make a list of everyone you can think of who might be a source of support. Include anyone who you think could help, even if you are not sure. List friends, relatives, work colleagues, and neighbors. Don't forget clergy, doctors, therapists or community agencies; include long-distance friends and online chat room buddies too. When you are finished, group the names according to the type of support they may provide. Remember, some people may be in more than one group. Keep this list handy—it is your support directory.

Step Two: Evaluate Your Needs

Now that you understand the types of social support and have thought about the people in your life who might provide you with that support, take a moment to reflect on your needs. The type of support you need will vary at different times in your life. If you are pregnant, you may need someone to talk to about what to expect in the months to come. If you have just delivered, you may need help with cooking or cleaning. If you have a toddler, you might need someone to babysit while you run a few errands. Consider what your needs may be at this time. And don't be shy about it! Feel free to include any support that you might wish for, even if it feels like a lot to ask.

Exercise: Identify Your Social Support Needs

Use the checklist below to identify any needs you have at this time. Make a check mark next to any item that you feel would help you. Don't worry if you don't see one of your needs listed here. Everyone has different needs, so we've left space for you to write in your own.

Emotional Support Needs

☐ Someone to listen to me

☐ Someone to talk with me about how it feels to be pregnant or a mother

☐ Reminders of my strengths

☐ Hugs or other physical affection

☐ Encouragement about how I'm doing as a new mom

☐ Empathy about how difficult pregnancy or motherhood can be

☐ _____

☐ _____

☐ _____

Practical Support Needs

☐ Help cooking meals

☐ Someone to babysit so I can have a break

☐ Assistance with laundry or other household tasks

☐ Someone to go to medical appointments with me

☐ Help with grocery shopping or errands

☐ Someone to hold the baby while I take a shower

☐ _____

☐ _____

☐ _____

Informational Support Needs

☐ Help making decisions about childcare

☐ Information about how to handle a newborn's sleep or other behavior issues

☐ Someone to show or tell me how to do things

☐ Assistance with planning labor and delivery strategies

☐ Information on how to handle common childhood illnesses, like colds or ear infections

☐ Help with breastfeeding

☐ _____

☐ _____

☐ _____

Peer Support Needs

☐ Hearing that others have had difficulty with pregnancy or motherhood too

☐ Hearing that breastfeeding gets easier

☐ Stories of children eventually sleeping through the night

☐ Strategies others have used to cope with difficult phases

☐ _____

☐ _____

☐ _____

Step Three: Challenge Unsupportive Thoughts

So now you know what you need and you know whom to ask, so why haven't you done it yet? If you are like many women, you may be reluctant to ask for help from others. Supermom myths and the pressure to do it all can keep you from getting the valuable support that you need. In this step, we'll review the skills you learned in chapter 5 and challenge any distorted thoughts that may keep you from asking for help. We've listed a few common ones below. Take a look and ask yourself whether you ever have the following thoughts:

- "I should be able to do everything myself."

- "I don't want to be a burden to others."

- "My baby's needs come first; mine are not important."

- "Asking for help makes me a weak person."

- "No one will want to help."

- "I should be able to fix this myself."

- "Others will think I'm selfish if I ask them to help."

- "Paying attention to my needs takes away from my time with my child."

- "Taking care of my baby is solely my responsibility."

- "My life should revolve around my child."

- "I don't have time to talk about my feelings or needs; there's too much to do."

Do you see yourself in any of these thoughts? If so, it is time to get to work. These thoughts are distorted and unfair, and they will keep you from getting the assistance you need. And not getting the support you need will keep you from being the best mom you can be.

For example, Belinda had the misperception that no one would want to take time out of their busy schedules to help her with her twin babies. So, even though she was struggling, she resisted asking any of her friends or relatives for assistance. So how did Belinda overcome her reluctance to tap into her network for some much-needed support? She used the technique of "conducting an experiment" (see chapter 5) to challenge this idea. She called up the members of her immediate family—her mom, sister, and brother—and tested out her theory by asking each of them if they'd be willing to come and visit her for a few days to help with the kids. To her surprise, everyone said yes! They didn't even hesitate—they were excited to meet the twins. Before she knew it, Belinda had two weeks' worth of visitors scheduled to come and help with the babies.

Remember Catherine's belief that she should be able to work at her usual high level of productivity despite the disruptive physical symptoms of pregnancy she was experiencing? She used the "examine the evidence" and "double standard" strategies described in chapter 5 to challenge her distorted thought. In doing so, she recalled colleagues who had decreased their hours during pregnancy, some others who had taken medical leave, and yet others whose billable hours decreased during times of personal difficulty. She realized that if a friend were in the same boat she would likely tell her that everyone has peaks and valleys in their job performance, that she has always been an exemplary employee, and that setbacks are common and expected. These strategies helped Catherine to change her distorted thought and allowed her to gain the courage to speak with her boss about temporarily reducing her hours during this tough time.

> ## Exercise: Challenge Your Unsupportive Thoughts
>
> Now you try it. Use the techniques we described in chapter 5 to challenge any distorted thoughts you may have about asking for help from others. Work to eliminate any ideas that your needs aren't a priority, that you should be able to juggle it all, or that others won't want to help you. Doing so will clear the way for you to get support during this challenging time.

Step Four: Ask for the Help You Need

The hardest part of getting your needs met can be the simple act of asking someone for their help. If you've challenged any thoughts that might have been obstacles to your support but you are still having trouble approaching others to ask for assistance, you may find this step particularly helpful. Remember, it is good for you and better for your baby when your needs are met.

To make sure you address those important needs, you may need some practice with a skill called *assertiveness*. Sometimes people worry that being assertive is the same as being aggressive, rude, or demanding. This is a common confusion. In fact, assertiveness is different from aggressiveness. Assertiveness means getting your needs met while respecting the rights of others.

With some practice, you can learn the art of assertive communication. You may feel strange doing this at first, but if you stick with it you'll become more comfortable expressing yourself, asking for the help you need, and, in the process, removing stress from your life.

Catherine practiced assertive communication by using the following steps to talk to her boss about decreasing her hours at work:

1. Choose the right person, time, and place. Try to pick a time when you and the other person are not angry, sleepy, or busy. Catherine knew she needed to speak to her supervisor to get her request approved and decided to set a meeting with him on the first Friday of the month, when things at the office tended to a be little calmer.

2. Express your feelings. Use "I" statements that say how you feel about the situation without blaming the other person. Catherine was able to tell her boss that, in her current situation, she did not feel able to perform her job at a level that met her high standards.

3. Make a specific request. Be specific and firm, but don't state it as an order. Catherine said that she wanted to decrease her work hours by 25 percent for the remainder of her pregnancy. She also made it clear that she would like to continue this schedule for at least three months following her maternity leave.

4. Outline the consequences. Be sure to outline the consequences of this new arrangement. Catherine was able to note the likely positive results of this new arrangement: her quality of work and morale would improve, and the firm would retain a valued and seasoned employee.

Exercise: Ask for Support

Now it's your turn. Pick a need from your list and then choose a person from your support directory who you think would be able to help you with that need. Using the steps above, ask that person for their assistance. You may be pleasantly surprised at the results and the positive impact that using your social support network has on your anxiety and your life.

Step Five: Improve Your Support Network

Even if you are working hard and doing the exercises we've outlined, you may have trouble getting the help you need if your support directory is thin. Or you may have a great group of supports but find that you have trouble getting aid in your particular areas of need. Whatever the case, it can never hurt to bolster your network of support. This allows you to choose your sources of support wisely and keeps you from making too many repeated requests of the same people.

Given your busy schedule as a pregnant or new mom, you may have to be creative in order to add new people to your support directory. Put on your thinking cap and brainstorm about options in your community, or use these ideas as a starting point:

- Join a new moms group

- Attend events or classes with your child at the local community center

- Start or join a play group

- Make an effort to call old friends you've lost touch with

- Go to a PTA meeting if you have children in elementary school

- Ask about babysitting services at local gyms or YMCAs

- Offer to trade favors, like babysitting, with other moms in your neighborhood

- Volunteer in your community and take your baby with you

- Log on to discussion boards for moms on websites such as www.babycenter.com

- Look for services in your community for new moms

- Check out websites like www.womenshealth.gov to learn about more about your health

Exercise: Build Your Support Network

Start with the list above and begin researching options for building your support network. Be creative. Ask friends, family, or neighbors for ideas too. Then go and do it! Pick one thing each week to try, and watch your support network blossom.

Next Steps

If you have tried the steps in this chapter and have opened the door for others to help you during this wonderful, yet challenging, time, congratulations! If, however, you are still having trouble getting the support you need, take a look back through the steps and see if anything in particular is tripping you up. Do you still have distorted thoughts about asking for help? Have you really considered *all* of your social support options? Did you practice making requests of others? Have you tried to expand your social support network? If you haven't tried all of these techniques, revisit these steps and keep practicing. Don't give up until you get the support that you need. Remember, families function best when all members are healthy, happy, and well cared for. You can be a good role model for your child by showing him or her that everyone's needs are important and should be respected. It may be hard, but keep trying! And, of course, if you are really stuck, talk to your obstetrician about support options in your community that might help.

Key Points

- Social support is integral to your health, particularly during pregnancy and the postpartum period.

- There are several types of social support, and the different people in your life may have strengths in different areas.

- Identifying your support people and your needs will help get you on the path toward good social support.

- If, like many women, you have trouble asking for help, challenging distorted thoughts will make it easier.

- There are many ways to expand your social support network. Check out choices in your community and build a healthy support system.

CHAPTER 13

Prevent Relapse

Feeling better is an amazing thing. Reducing your anxiety is hard work, and there's no better reward than watching the storm clouds lift and seeing the sun come out again. Finally, you can relax and enjoy your life. You don't feel as tense and on edge as you did before. Your obsessive thoughts no longer trouble you and your compulsions are long gone. Panic attacks have nearly vanished and your worry is under control. You no longer avoid things, your relationships are better, and you're more productive. In other words, you've defeated your anxiety problem.

You now know that overcoming anxiety requires learning and practicing specific techniques. And now that you've mastered the keys to overcoming anxiety, there's one more thing you need to know: how to stop it from happening again. In this chapter, we'll show you the essentials of preventing the return of anxiety:

- How we define a relapse

- The keys to preventing a relapse

- What to do if you have another child

- What to do if you need additional help

What Is a Relapse?

Before he would talk about any important topic, the Greek philosopher Socrates insisted on defining the terms that would be used in the discussion. So, before we talk about relapse, let's start by defining the term. What exactly does it mean to have a "relapse"? Researchers and clinicians may use many different definitions, but in our practice we believe you've suffered a relapse if any symptom of anxiety has returned and is significantly interfering with your life.

Let's also talk about what we don't consider a relapse. Every client that we treat for anxiety inevitably experiences some anxiety symptoms again. In fact, it's safe to say that every person on this planet will experience anxiety from time to time. So, whether you've had obsessive thoughts, or worry, or panic attacks or any of the other anxiety problems listed in this book, it's likely you'll have them again. The good news is that feeling anxious at times doesn't mean you've relapsed—it just means you're human. To find out if you're having a relapse, ask yourself whether your anxiety symptoms disrupt your life in some meaningful and important way. If the answer is yes, then we would consider that a relapse.

For example, let's suppose you picked up this book because you were suffering from panic attacks that started during your pregnancy. You worked hard and applied the strategies described in this book. Some helped; some didn't. Over time and with practice, you slowly lessened your panic attacks and regained control of your life. You've been panic free for weeks now. Once you avoided things like driving and shopping; now you do these things with comfort and ease. You are truly enjoying life again. In fact, you feel so good you wonder if you'll ever have another panic attack.

Then, one day while walking your new daughter in the stroller, you have that uneasy feeling again. Your heart starts to beat faster, your breath quickens, and your palms start to sweat. It feels like you might be having a heart attack or going crazy. The next thing you know, you're having a full-blown panic attack. A few minutes pass and the panic fades. You feel better. You think, "That was weird. I haven't felt that way in a while." And you go on with your leisurely walk—and your life.

Does having that panic attack mean you've relapsed? Luckily, it doesn't. One panic attack does not constitute a relapse. In order to meet our criteria for a relapse, your anxiety symptoms have to be so intense that they disrupt your life in some way.

Let's look at the experience of Lilly, a new mom we treated recently who did have an anxiety relapse. Lilly initially came to therapy because she started experiencing obsessive thoughts of harming her three-month-old daughter, Riley. Lilly was particularly troubled by a recurrent intrusive image of smothering her daughter with a pillow. Lilly had developed a compulsion to cope with her harming obsession—she avoided putting her daughter to bed at night and had her husband do it instead.

Within a few weeks of starting therapy, which involved using the techniques described in this book, Lilly felt much better. After just a few more sessions, she was ready to terminate therapy. Her obsessions no longer troubled her and she now looked forward to putting her daughter to bed each night. She even felt comfortable enough to do it alone.

About six months after she had ended therapy, Lilly called to make another appointment. During that appointment she stated that she'd faced her harming obsessions many more times since her last session, and she now felt she had the tools to manage them. However, Lilly was struggling with a new obsession, a fear that she would transmit a horrible disease to her daughter, and was feeling stuck. Although she was nowhere near as anxious as she had been before, she still felt trapped and didn't know how to get out. In addition, her new

> ## ~ COMMON QUESTION ~
> ### If I relapse, will I have the same problem or a different one?
>
> Now that you're feeling better, you might wonder if you'll have the same anxiety symptoms again in the future, or if you'll be faced with a new anxiety challenge. Unfortunately, it's tough to say. For some people, the same problem rears its head again and again. They have to remain extra vigilant to that specific problem and be consistent in practicing the techniques to manage it. Other people find that they conquer one anxiety problem only to face a new one in the future. Either way, it can be helpful for you to familiarize yourself with the other anxiety symptoms described in this book so you'll know what they are and how you can overcome them.

obsession was causing her to wash her hands excessively and avoid certain activities, like eating out at restaurants and using public restrooms. Because Lilly's new obsession was disrupting her life in a significant way, we would say that Lilly had relapsed. Fortunately, it took just a few more sessions of practicing some additional techniques for Lilly to get back to her old self again.

Your Personal Relapse Prevention Plan

Now that you understand what it means to have a relapse, you're ready to create your personal relapse prevention plan. There are five keys to your relapse prevention plan:

1. Know your warning signs

2. Know what worked for you in the past

3. Keep practicing

4. Rewrite your anxiety rule book

5. Make healthy lifestyle changes

Step One: Know Your Warning Signs

One of the first steps you can take to stop a relapse in its tracks is to know the *warning signs* of a relapse. Like a smoke detector that sounds at the first sign of a fire, a warning sign is an early signal of a recurrence of your anxiety problem.

There are three different types of warning signs:

- The consistent presence of anxiety symptoms

- Signs that anxiety is interfering with your life

- The occurrence of stressful events in your life

One of the first warning signs of a relapse is the continuing presence of anxiety symptoms in your life. As we stated earlier, the occasional anxiety symptom—such as a panic attack or an intrusive thought—is part of being human, much like the occasional headache or bad mood. However, if you notice that you're repeatedly bothered by one or more of the symptoms described in this book, then that may be a sign that your anxiety problem is starting to take root again.

It's also important, as you work on preventing a relapse, to be alert for signs that anxiety is interfering with your life; often, these signs start small. For many people, one of the first signs of a relapse is avoidance. People often report that they had been fully engaged in life but as the anxiety set back in they started avoiding certain places and activities again. Avoidance is a clear sign that anxiety is running your life. If you catch yourself relying on avoidance to manage your anxiety, make a mental note—it may be a key sign that you're in danger of having a relapse.

The last warning sign is the presence of stressful events in your life that may trigger a relapse. Of course, life in general is stressful, but life with a newborn can be particularly taxing as you cope with crying, feeding, and disrupted sleep. Other stressful events can include moving, job changes, or arguments with your significant other. As you look back on your life, you might note specific events that you found particularly stressful. Maybe arguing with your spouse or financial strain hits you especially hard. Your trigger might even be "good" stress, such as a promotion or buying a house. Whatever your triggers are, it's crucial to be aware of them and prepare for them as a potential cause of a future relapse.

Exercise: What Are Your Warning Signs?

Below you'll find warning signs, grouped in the form of anxiety symptoms, signs of interference from anxiety, and stressful events. Read through each group and identify your warning signs of a relapse.

Anxiety Symptoms

Check off any of the following anxiety symptoms that you've had in the past or that you have been experiencing in the present:

- ☐ Panic attacks
- ☐ Obsessions
- ☐ Compulsions
- ☐ Worry
- ☐ Post-traumatic stress
- ☐ Other _____

Signs Anxiety Is Interfering with Your Life

Now, identify any signs of anxiety interfering with your life. Make a check mark next to any signs that you've experienced in the past or that you think you might experience in the future:

- ☐ Avoidance
- ☐ Withdrawal
- ☐ Procrastination
- ☐ Substance use or abuse
- ☐ Reassurance seeking
- ☐ Worry behaviors (checking, repeating, superstitions)

☐ Physical symptoms (headache, backache, upset stomach, insomnia)

☐ Emotional symptoms (depression, anger, anxiety)

☐ Interpersonal symptoms (irritability, avoidance of intimacy, dependency on others)

☐ Lifestyle changes (poor eating habits, lack of exercise)

☐ Other signs of interference _____

Stressful Events

Now place a check mark next to specific triggers that have caused you anxiety in the past or that you think might cause anxiety in the future:

☐ Relationship discord

☐ Job stress (arguments with your boss, layoffs, demotion)

☐ Financial stress (unexpected bills, taking on debt, stopping work)

☐ Illness (in yourself, your family, others)

☐ Social isolation

☐ Major life changes (moving, new job)

☐ Legal problems

☐ Relationship problems (with family, friends, coworkers)

☐ Loss of a loved one

☐ Other triggers _____

Step Two: Know What Worked for You

Now that you've identified your warning signs of a relapse, take a moment to reflect on the exercises in this book. All of them are effective ways to treat anxiety, but not all of them work for everyone. Overcoming anxiety is a trial-and-error process. Like our clients, you probably have your favorite techniques, the ones that were the most helpful to you. Perhaps you found the relaxation techniques to be especially useful. Maybe the cognitive methods helped you banish your anxiety. Or maybe it was a combination of techniques that worked.

Whatever methods you found useful, those techniques are crucial to preventing a relapse. They are like your personal anxiety tool kit. They are the strategies that you can use over and over. Best of all, unlike prescription medication, they don't have an expiration date.

Exercise: What Worked for You?

Use the checklist below to identify the exercises that worked for you. Place a check mark next to any technique that was helpful, even if it only helped a bit.

Relaxation Strategies

☐ PMR

☐ Diaphragmatic breathing

☐ Guided imagery

☐ Other relaxing activities (such as massage and yoga)

Modifying Anxious Thoughts

☐ Identify anxious thoughts

☐ Identify cognitive distortions

☐ Examine the evidence

☐ Generate alternatives

☐ Anticatastrophic thinking

☐ Double standard

☐ Image substitution

☐ Conduct an experiment

☐ Talk to other moms

Exposure and Response Prevention Techniques

☐ Real-life exposure

☐ Imaginal exposure

☐ Physical symptom exposure

☐ Response prevention

Problem Solving and Planning

☐ Problem-solving skills

☐ Time management

Warning Signs and Techniques: Putting It All Together

Transfer the information from the checklists above to the form below. This will give you all the information you need to spot a relapse and stop it in its tracks.

1. The anxiety symptoms that I need to watch out for are the following:

    _____

    _____

    _____

2. I know anxiety is interfering with my life when:

    _____

    _____

    _____

3. The stressful life events that tend to trigger my anxiety are:

    _____

    _____

    _____

4. The techniques that most help me control my anxiety are:

    _____

    _____

    _____

Step Three: Keep Up Your Practice

Once you've overcome your anxiety problem, it can be tempting to put all of this behind you, forget you ever had these symptoms, and move on with your life. After all, as a new mom, you now have responsibilities and pressures that were impossible to imagine just a short time ago.

However, to maintain your progress and prevent a relapse, you need to keep up your practice with the techniques described in this book. It's the same with exercise: just like you wouldn't stop exercising once you'd gotten in shape, you need to keep working on controlling your anxiety even though you're feeling better.

Of course, for a new mom or mom-to-be, finding time to practice can be especially difficult. It can be helpful to set aside a specific time each week that you'll use to work on managing your anxiety.

Consider this "therapy time," and schedule it just like you would a regular therapy appointment. Look back at the exercise titled What Worked for You? and practice those techniques during your therapy time. Remember, regular practice goes a long way toward preventing a relapse.

Step Four: Rewrite Your Anxiety Rule Book

Throughout this book, we've showed you specific techniques that address the symptoms of anxiety. We've given you a straightforward model for helping yourself to feel better: identify your symptoms and then apply certain techniques to make those symptoms go away.

Like many of our clients, though, you might wonder how you came to have this anxiety problem in the first place. One way to peer a bit deeper into your anxiety problem is to examine some of the rules you've developed that guide you through life—your "anxiety rule book." The anxiety rule book consists of your core beliefs that make you vulnerable to anxiety. These beliefs make you vulnerable to anxiety now and in the future. Even though everyone is different, these rules tend to be consistent from person to person for each anxiety problem.

Let's suppose you picked up this book because you were worrying too much. After using some of the techniques in this book, you feel your worry is much more under control. However, if we were to look at your anxiety rule book, we might find that you still hold the belief "Worry helps me. If I don't worry, something bad might happen." This belief can be considered a rule for living: when things get rough, worry. As you can imagine, even after you've used the strategies in this book, if you keep this belief as part of your rule book, you'll be much more vulnerable to a relapse in the future.

If you're going to make long-term changes, it's crucial that you rewrite your anxiety rule book. By changing your rule book, you'll protect yourself from relapse.

> **Exercise:** Rewrite Your Anxiety Rule Book.

Take a look at the old rules in the chart below. Do any of them sound familiar? If so, take a look at the new rules listed across from the old ones. Think about replacing your old rules with these newer, more flexible rules.

The Anxiety Rule Book	
Old Rules	**New Rules**
1. **Panic attacks:** If I feel bad in certain situations, I should avoid those situations. It's bad to feel bad. Feeling bad or weird is dangerous and means there's something wrong with me.	1. **Panic attacks:** I'll do what I need or want to do regardless of how I feel. Feeling bad or weird sometimes is normal and doesn't necessarily mean something is wrong with me.
2. **Obsessions:** My thoughts are really important and meaningful and I should try to control them. I need certainty.	2. **Obsessions:** Everyone has bad thoughts at times. They don't mean anything. I can accept the uncertainty inherent in life.

3. **Compulsions:** Doing this behavior will protect me or my child. It will prevent harm. I must do whatever I can to protect my children.

3. **Compulsions:** These compulsions really do nothing to reduce risk and only make me feel better in the short term. Doing this compulsion means I'll feel like I have to do it for the rest of my life—unless I stop now.

4. **Worry:** Worry helps me. If I don't worry I might miss something, or something bad might happen.

4. **Worry:** Productive worry can help if I use it to solve problems. Unproductive worry is a waste of time and energy.

5. **Post-traumatic stress:** I must always be on guard. I can't trust people. I can't let it happen again.

5. **Post-traumatic stress:** I'll be prudent, but it's okay to relax and enjoy my life. I can take smart risks.

Step Five: Make Healthy Lifestyle Changes

Although unhealthy lifestyle habits are rarely the cause of an anxiety problem, making healthy lifestyle changes can reduce the likelihood that you'll experience an anxiety problem again in the future. Lifestyle changes you can make that are particularly valuable to preventing a relapse include the following (McCabe and Antony 2005):

- Scheduling your time effectively
- Developing healthy sleep habits
- Modifying your diet
- Getting regular exercise

Let's take a look at these lifestyle changes one at a time.

Schedule Your Time Effectively

Having an anxiety problem, with all of the worrying, planning avoidance strategies, and doing compulsions, can take up a tremendous amount of time. When your anxiety decreases, you may find that you have more free time than you did before. Anxiety thrives on free time. It can be an enormous help to fill that time with more enjoyable and productive activities (Franklin, Riggs, and Pai 2005). Our anxious clients frequently tell us that when they are busy and distracted, they feel better.

One way to schedule your time effectively and reduce the likelihood of a relapse is to use a technique called *activity scheduling,* or purposefully planning activities to fill your free time. What kind of activities should you put in your schedule? There are two types of activities to consider: *pleasant* and *mastery* (Burns 1999).

As the name suggests, pleasant activities are those that you may find fun, pleasurable, or enjoyable. Here are some examples:

- ☐ Taking a bath
- ☐ Getting a massage
- ☐ Seeing a movie
- ☐ Listening to music
- ☐ Taking a walk
- ☐ Going out to dinner
- ☐ Talking to a friend
- ☐ Gardening

- ☐ Cooking a gourmet meal
- ☐ Doing a puzzle
- ☐ Hiking
- ☐ Taking a bike ride
- ☐ Going to the beach or a park
- ☐ Photography
- ☐ Playing a musical instrument

Mastery activities, on the other hand, are those activities that aren't necessarily fun but give us a sense of satisfaction or accomplishment. For example, most of us don't enjoy cleaning the bathroom. However, when it's done, we often feel satisfied and pleased. Mastery activities are often the things you put off when you procrastinate. Here are some other examples:

- ☐ Paying your bills
- ☐ Going to the dentist or doctor
- ☐ Balancing your checkbook
- ☐ Cleaning
- ☐ Writing thank-you notes
- ☐ Car maintenance or repairs

- ☐ Laundry or dry cleaning
- ☐ Making travel arrangements
- ☐ Reading unopened mail or responding to e-mail
- ☐ Studying
- ☐ Returning phone calls

Exercise: Select and Schedule Pleasant and Mastery Activities

Take out a sheet of paper and draw a line down the middle. On one side, write the heading "Pleasure," and on the other side write "Mastery." On the pleasure side, list activities that you've enjoyed—either currently or at some point in the past—or activities you think you'd enjoy but have never actually tried. On the mastery side, list chores and activities that give you a sense of accomplishment when completed. List anything you've been putting off, such as seeing your doctor or returning a phone call. Once you've listed activities that will bring you pleasure or a sense of mastery, plug these activities into slots in your day whenever you have free time. Try to schedule at least one activity each day.

Develop Healthy Sleep Habits

Poor sleep makes anxiety problems worse. When you're tired, you'll find that panic attacks occur more frequently, obsessive thoughts increase, compulsions are harder to fight, and you worry more. Getting a good night's rest on a regular basis can be a tremendous help in the battle against anxiety. Of course, with a newborn, fragmented sleep is part of the deal. However, you can take steps to improve your sleep habits and get the most out of your opportunities to sleep. These steps include the following:

1. Go to bed at around the same time every night. Try to get up around the same time each morning.

2. Avoid caffeine after four o'clock in the afternoon.

3. Use your bed only for sleeping and sex. Don't read or watch TV in bed.

4. Experiment with naps. When you have a newborn, napping when your baby naps is essential. When you are pregnant, you may need those naps to make it through your day. However, make sure naps don't interfere with your ability to fall asleep at night. If they do, consider avoiding them, moving them to earlier in the day, or shortening them.

5. Avoid exercising right before bed.

6. If you're unable to fall asleep within about twenty minutes after getting into bed, get up and do something boring in another room, like reading a dull book or balancing your checkbook. Get back into bed as soon as you feel sleepy again.

Modify Your Diet

Diet and exercise—we've all heard that before, right? But it's true—making even small changes to your diet and starting an exercise program can go a long way toward preventing a relapse. What diet changes can you make? As a new or expectant mother, you have specific dietary needs at this point in your life and we want you to follow the recommendations of your doctor. Beyond that, Dr. Susan Kleiner (Kleiner and Condor 2007), author of *The Good Mood Diet,* suggests eliminating problem foods such as fried foods, foods loaded with refined sugar, and caffeine. She also suggests adding calming, mood-enhancing foods such as nuts, fish, eggs, dairy, and fruits and vegetables.

Get Regular Exercise

Studies have shown that cardiovascular exercise is an effective way to manage anxiety and stress (Long and van Stavel 1995). Cardiovascular exercise burns off excess anxiety and stress and resets your stress response. Experts recommend getting about thirty minutes of cardiovascular exercise per day. Thankfully, evidence suggests that the thirty minutes don't have to happen all at once to generate the desired health benefits. Possible ways to get thirty minutes of cardio a day include the following:

- Taking the stairs

- Walking

- Biking

- Rollerblading

- Shoveling snow

- Jumping rope

- Dancing

- Swimming

- Jogging

Mom, meet your new personal trainer. As your newborn child grows and starts crawling and walking, you have a marvelous opportunity to have your own personal trainer. Unlike professional trainers, your little one is free, doesn't require an appointment, and probably won't take no for an answer. So capitalize on this opportunity to get active. Chase your baby around, play hide-and-seek, and wrestle. Build obstacle courses and climb them. Teach your child to ride a tricycle and run alongside. Climb slides at the park. Take your child sledding. Go for daily walks. Take your baby on bike rides. Put on some music and dance. As your baby grows up, teach her to ice skate and swim and ride a two-wheeler. Not only will you be building a lifelong connection with your child, you'll easily meet your goal of thirty minutes of cardio a day, and that'll go a long way toward preventing the return of your anxiety problem.

Should You Have Another Child?

One of the most common questions new moms ask us once they've conquered their anxiety is "Do you think I should have another child?" Of course, what they really mean is "Do you think I'll be okay if I have another child?"

Unfortunately, we don't have a crystal ball, so we can't predict the future. In addition, there's a lot more to factor into that decision than just anxiety, such as finances, lifestyle, and your family's needs and preferences. Having another child really is a personal choice. Our hope is that you've reduced your anxiety sufficiently so that it's not the deciding factor. We believe you should make that choice based on what you want, not based on fear.

> ### ~ COMMON QUESTION ~
> #### Will my next pregnancy be the same as this one?
>
> Unfortunately, there's no way to tell for sure. You might sail through your next pregnancy and postpartum scot-free. Or you might have a similar experience next time around. Or, it could be worse. There's really no way to know. As you read earlier in this book, pregnancy and the postpartum period can be a time when some anxiety symptoms escalate. However, that doesn't happen in all cases. In fact, some women seem even more relaxed as they enter into motherhood and experience a reprieve from their anxiety symptoms.

That being said, a preexisting anxiety problem is one of the best predictors of anxiety during pregnancy and postpartum. Therefore, if you've experienced anxiety symptoms during this pregnancy or postpartum period, it's likely that you'll experience anxiety symptoms again if you decide to have more children. Keep in mind, though, that you now have effective tools to manage your anxiety. Armed with this knowledge, you can more effectively address any symptoms that do arise and head them off at the pass.

Exercise: Conduct a Cost-Benefit Analysis

Having another child is often an emotional decision. It can seem cold to reduce it to a cost-benefit analysis. However, if you suffered from anxiety during this pregnancy or postpartum period, it can be useful to weigh the potential costs and benefits of having another child, so you can make a well-thought-out decision. Take out a sheet of paper and at the top write "Having another baby." Then draw a line down the middle and write "Costs" on the left and "Benefits" on the right. List all the drawbacks of having another child, including the possibility of experiencing anxiety again. Then list all the benefits. Which side is more convincing?

If You Need Additional Help

If, after working on the solutions described in this book, you find that anxiety is still a significant problem for you, it might benefit you to seek additional help. Finding a therapist trained in cognitive behavioral therapy and experienced with anxiety disorders could be the key to change. Professional organizations such as the Anxiety Disorders Association of America (www.adaa.org), the Association of Behavioral and Cognitive Therapies (www.abct.org), and the Academy of Cognitive Therapy (www.academyofct.org) can help you find a qualified therapist in your area.

Final Words

For us—psychologists who treat anxiety problems—seeing our anxious clients improve is the zenith of our work. There's no better moment in our workday than when our clients tell us, "I feel great!" When we work hard together and our clients finally feel relief, it's like they've climbed Mount Everest. And we've had a front-row seat for the climb, so we get to momentarily enjoy the view with them.

These moments can be a bit bittersweet, though, because we know that all of our clients, no matter how hard they've worked, will experience some form of anxiety again. We hope that the anxiety they—and you—experience in the future doesn't become a full-blown relapse. Remember that the key to understanding and preventing relapse is to know exactly what you need to do if you do have these symptoms again. Should you suffer a relapse, in most cases the best approach is to apply the same solutions that worked for you the first time. If these strategies worked once, it's likely that they'll work again. All you need to do is add the time and effort.

Key Points

- We define a relapse as a return of anxiety symptoms at a high enough level that they significantly interfere with your life.

- Effective relapse prevention consists of five key steps: knowing your warning signs, knowing what worked for you in the past, continuing to practice your skills, rewriting your anxiety rule book, and making healthy lifestyle changes.

- If you're considering having another child, factor in the potential for increased anxiety. But also consider other aspects, such as your personal values, lifestyle, and preferences. And remember that you now have effective tools to manage your anxiety.

- If you suffer a relapse and can't seem to get unstuck, consider seeking professional help from a psychologist or psychiatrist trained in treating anxiety problems.

CHAPTER 14

For Dads Only: How to Cope with Fatherhood & Support Your Partner

If you're a new or expectant dad who is suffering from feelings of depression or anxiety, or if your partner is struggling with these feelings and you're wondering how you can best help her, this chapter is for you. We've divided this chapter into two parts. In part 1, we'll describe common difficulties that men experience as they become fathers, and we'll give you specific strategies for coping with these problems. In part 2, we'll identify key ways you can help your partner cope with the emotional challenges of becoming a mom.

What You Might Experience

Whether you're a new dad or a dad-to-be, you probably already realize something about fatherhood: it's the highest of the highs—and the lowest of the lows. You're on an emotional roller coaster unlike any you'll ever experience. One moment, you're beaming, the proud dad of a beautiful newborn. The next, you're swamped with worry, wondering how you'll make ends meet, get enough sleep, or just have an adult conversation with your partner. It is truly a time of incredible joy and unbelievable stress. Unfortunately, all the stress that surrounds parenthood—from sleepless nights to the cost of diapers—makes it a time when you are particularly vulnerable to painful emotions such as depression and anxiety. No one knows this better than John.

When his son, Evan, was born, John was in the delivery room holding his wife's hand. As the doctors tended to his wife, a nurse gently handed John his new son and brought them to the recovery room. There, John spent a few minutes alone with Evan. Wearing blue scrubs, John sat in a wheelchair, cradling his beautiful son, and wept with joy. He thought of all the wonders that lay ahead—fishing together, playing catch in the yard, teaching his son to drive. A photographer at the hospital took a picture of Evan, and John slipped it into his wallet.

Unfortunately, John's initial feelings of joy didn't last. Even though he loved Evan dearly and becoming a father was a dream come true, fatherhood hit John hard. Shortly after Evan's birth, John noticed that he didn't feel right. Despite being exhausted, he couldn't sleep. He couldn't focus at work. He felt irritable, ready to snap at the slightest provocation. He lost his appetite and he lost weight. Nothing felt fun or interesting anymore. At times, John even thought of taking his own life. John was suffering from postpartum depression.

Dads and Postpartum Depression

Like John, you might be surprised to learn that men can suffer from postpartum depression. Once thought to affect only women, postpartum depression is now known to be common in men as well. Recently, researchers at Eastern Virginia Medical School found that, following the birth of a child, 10 percent of men suffer emotional symptoms severe enough to meet criteria for depression (Paulson, Dauber, and Leiferman 2006).

If you're suffering from depression following the birth of your child, you'll be experiencing some or all of the common symptoms of depression. According to the American Psychiatric Association (2000), these symptoms include the following:

- Depressed or sad mood

- Loss of interest in activities

- Significant weight loss or weight gain

- Difficulty sleeping or sleeping too much

- Fatigue or loss of energy

- Strong feelings of guilt or worthlessness

- Difficulty concentrating or trouble making decisions

- Thoughts of death or suicide

Everyone experiences some of these symptoms from time to time. For example, if you're a new dad, you'll certainly feel fatigued, be lacking in energy, and have difficulty concentrating at times. If you have several of these symptoms, though, and they don't resolve over time, you may be suffering from depression.

> ~ COMMON QUESTION ~
> **What might make me vulnerable to depression?**
>
> No one is sure why some dads suffer from depression and others don't. However, there are some clear risk factors. For example, postpartum depression and anxiety in your partner is a significant risk factor in your becoming depressed. In fact, studies show that up to 50 percent of men with a partner who is suffering from postpartum depression are depressed as well (Lovestone and Kumar 1993). If you have a history of depression, you may also be more likely to experience depression after the birth of your child. Therefore, if your partner is currently depressed or if you have a history of depression, be particularly watchful for symptoms of depression as you become a dad.

When Does Depression in Fathers Usually Start?

While you might find the weeks immediately following the birth of your child to be the most stressful time, depression can strike at any time, including during your partner's pregnancy and well into the first year of your child's life.

Anxiety in Dads During Pregnancy and the Postpartum Period

Anxiety is another common problem that men experience during pregnancy and postpartum. The most common anxiety symptoms that you might experience include the following:

- Panic attacks

- Worry

- Obsessive thoughts

- Compulsions

Let's look at more-detailed descriptions of each of these potential problems.

Panic Attacks

Panic attacks are sudden rushes of intense anxiety that usually last ten to fifteen minutes. During these attacks, you might feel like you're having a heart attack, going crazy, or about to die. While panic attacks are generally harmless, they can be frightening. They can also disrupt your life if they happen frequently (such as several times a day) or cause you to avoid activities or situations, such as driving, flying, or crowded places.

Worry

Worry is simply catastrophic thinking about the future. You can usually tell if you're worrying when you notice that you have a "what if" thought followed by a "Something bad is going to happen" type of thought. For example, you might think, "What if my son gets sick and dies?" Or, "What if I don't save enough for college and I can't afford to send my son to school?" If you're prone to worry, you might also worry about things like the health of your baby, your finances, or your marriage. Chronic worry often leads to unpleasant physical symptoms, such as muscle tension, headaches, or fatigue (American Psychiatric Association 2000).

Obsessions

An obsession is an unwanted, intrusive thought that causes significant anxiety or distress. The pregnancy and postpartum period may be a time when fathers are particularly vulnerable to obsessive thoughts (Abramowitz et al. 2001). Though you might experience any kind of obsessive thought, certain themes are particularly common for new parents:

- **Violent obsessions:** These obsessive thoughts can include thoughts of harm coming to your child or you directly causing harm to your child. For example, if you have obsessions about harming your child, you might have unwanted thoughts of stabbing him while you're feeding him a bottle or thoughts of drowning him while you're giving him a bath.

- **Sexual obsessions:** As the name suggests, sexual obsessions are intrusive thoughts of sexually molesting your child. While these types of thoughts are common, they can cause intense anxiety, especially during parenting activities that involve close contact with your newborn, such as changing diapers, giving baths, or dressing your baby.

Note: While violent or sexual obsessions can be frightening, they are common, especially during the postpartum period. It's important to note that these thoughts are usually harmless. However, if you're concerned that you might act on them, please discuss them with your doctor or a mental health professional. You can also read more about these thoughts in chapter 9.

> ~ COMMON QUESTION ~
> ### What if I have both obsessions and compulsions?
>
> Obsessions and compulsions almost always go together, and certain pairings of the two are common. For example, if you have obsessions about contamination, it's likely that you'll compulsively wash or clean. On the other hand, if you experience violent or sexual obsessions, you might rely more on avoidance or reassurance seeking as a compulsion.

- **Contamination obsessions:** Fears of contaminating yourself or someone you love, such as your wife or baby, are among the most common obsessions. If you have contamination obsessions, you might fear contracting a horrible illness, like AIDS. In turn, with a newborn baby in your house, you'll feel an intense responsibility to protect your child, and you might fear that you could transmit this illness to her.

Compulsions

Compulsions are repetitive behaviors whose main purpose is to reduce anxiety. Examples of compulsions include checking your sleeping baby frequently to make sure she's still breathing, washing or cleaning excessively, or repeatedly seeking reassurance that your baby is safe and healthy. You might rely also on avoidance as a compulsion to reduce your distress. For example, if you have violent or sexual obsessions, you might refuse to spend time alone with your baby because of your fear that you'll harm her in some way.

Eight Keys to Coping Well

If you're suffering from any of the symptoms above, there are some important steps you can take to change how you feel. For dads, it's part of the job description to suffer from sleep deprivation, spit-up-stained clothes, and a sore back. It's not necessary, however, to suffer from depression or anxiety. Below, we've listed eight keys to coping with the stresses and strains of fatherhood.

1. Use This Book

In part 2 of this book, we describe specific techniques you can use to conquer anxiety. These methods include relaxation training, cognitive restructuring, exposure exercises, and response prevention. If you're experiencing any symptoms of anxiety, including panic attacks, worry, obsessive thoughts, or compulsions, you can use these techniques to manage your symptoms. For help with applying these techniques to specific symptoms, refer to part 3 of this book, where we describe the steps for overcoming panic, obsessions, and other anxiety symptoms using the methods illustrated in part 2.

2. Consider the Benefits of Fatherhood

After getting up in the middle of the night for the fifth time to soothe your crying baby, you might wonder, "Why did I do this? Why did I voluntarily choose to give up sleep, sanity, and regular sex? What's the matter with me? What was I thinking?" Those sleep-deprived moments prove Bill Cosby (1987) right when he said, "Yes, having a child is surely the most beautifully irrational act that two people in love can commit."

Nevertheless, you did get into this for a reason. As you struggle with never-ending diaper changes, a cranky spouse, and meddling in-laws, it can be tremendously helpful to recall the reasons you chose to have a child. You might think about the more immediate payoffs like seeing your son smile for the first time, or far-off rewards such as hugging your daughter after she graduates from college.

List the benefits of being a father that are especially meaningful to you in the space below:

_____

_____

_____

_____

_____

Be sure to review this list often. These reasons might be just the things that pull you through the tough times.

3. Generate Coping Statements

Psychologists have known for a long time that what you say to yourself has a profound impact on how you feel. This is definitely true when it comes to fatherhood. The good news is that you can use this knowledge to your advantage by creating your own coping statements to help you through the dark moments. Even professional athletes use this method to cope with the stress of competition. As a parent, you can also use this technique to feel more calm and relaxed. For example, researchers

(McKay, Rogers, and McKay 2003) noted that parents who reported less distress while parenting used specific coping statements to help lessen their stress. You can use coping statements as well to help you manage your own negative feelings. Here are some examples to consider:

- "He's just a child. He doesn't know any better."

- "She isn't trying to upset me; she is just trying to get what she wants."

- "This is normal behavior for a child his age."

- "She is probably hungry or tired."

- "I can cope with this. I'm the adult here. I am in control."

Dan used this technique to successfully manage the feelings of anxiety and stress that plagued him when he was caring for his new daughter, Sydney. He identified his daughter's crying as a situation that was especially upsetting to him. Then he recorded several coping statements on an index card. He included thoughts such as "She's an infant. She doesn't know any better," and "She's not trying to upset me. She's too young for that." Then, when his negative feelings became too strong, he pulled out his card and reviewed these coping statements to ease his feelings of anxiety and stress.

You can use this technique to manage your own negative feelings. In the spaces below, write five coping thoughts that you can use to help you manage your own feelings of stress and anxiety:

1. _____

2. _____

3. _____

4. _____

5. _____

Be sure to do this when you have some quiet, uninterrupted time. Later, when the spit-up starts flying and the anxiety starts rising, you can review these thoughts to help calm yourself down.

4. Get Support

Being a dad can be a lonely, isolating experience. You might feel like a lone soldier in battle, coping with the stress of fatherhood, knee-deep in diapers, in over your head. In order to preserve your sanity, you need to tap into a network of social support. Potential sources of support include the following:

- Your spouse or significant other

- Your mother and/or father

- Siblings

- Friends

- Coworkers

- Other new dads

- More-experienced dads

- Childbirth classes

- Clergy or other spiritual resources

- Therapists

Since support is so crucial to a person's ability to cope with the stress of parenting, take a moment and list your main sources of assistance and advice:

1. _____

2. _____

3. _____

4. _____

5. _____

Now that you've identified your main support people, be sure you schedule time to get together or talk with them regularly. Finding time for this may take more effort with a new child in your life, so you'll have to be proactive and plan in advance when you'll see them. The benefits—enjoying a better mood, feeling less isolated, regaining a sense of balance—will be well worth it.

5. Get Some Sleep

It's easier said than done, right? Disrupted sleep is a rite of passage for new dads. However, if you're suffering from postpartum depression or anxiety, getting some rest is one of the most important things you can do. Studies have shown that sleep plays a key role in lessening postpartum depression in moms (Armstrong et al. 1998). There's no reason to think dads are any different. So put getting enough sleep at the top of your priority list.

If you're having trouble sleeping, try the following tips:

- Go to bed at the same time every night and get up at the same time each morning.

- Avoid caffeine after four o'clock in the afternoon.

- Use your bed only for sleeping and sex. Don't read or watch TV in bed.

- Experiment with naps. When you have a newborn, napping when your baby naps is essential. However, make sure your naps don't interfere with your ability to fall asleep at night.

- Avoid exercising right before bed.

- If you're unable to fall asleep within twenty minutes after getting into bed, get up and do something boring in another room, like reading a dull book or balancing your checkbook. Get back into bed as soon as you feel sleepy again.

6. Boost Your Skills

Maybe you have a fantastic role model who has shown you how to be a great dad. If so, consider yourself lucky, because the truth is this: no one is born knowing how to parent. And that nagging sense that you don't know what you're doing is a major contributor to feelings of anxiety and depression. Fortunately, there's no lack of resources to help you enhance your skills and feel more confident. Here are some specific ways to improve your parenting skills:

- Read a few respected parenting books or magazines.

- Attend parenting classes.

- Visit parenting websites for information and ideas.

- Seek advice from fathers you admire.

- Exchange tips and ideas with other new fathers.

- Discuss child-rearing issues with your pediatrician.

7. Know That Dads Matter

In the last few decades, there's been a dramatic shift in the role that fathers play in raising their children. Dads are no longer taking a backseat to moms in child-care decisions. The difference is visible. Go to any park, kid-friendly restaurant, or mall and you'll see dads out in force changing diapers, playing peek-a-boo, and giving bottles.

Spending time with their dads is clearly a good thing for kids. In fact, a wealth of compelling research highlights just how critical a father is to his child's development. First, a high level of father involvement provides cognitive and emotional benefits. In a study of preschool-aged children, those whose fathers were responsible for 40 percent or more of the child-care tasks had higher cognitive development scores, more of a sense of mastery of their environment, and more empathy than those with less-involved fathers (Radin 1994).

Second, involvement by fathers seems to lessen the occurrence of children's emotional problems. One study found that fathers who get involved when their children at an early age had children who experienced fewer emotional problems and distress during adolescence and adulthood (Flouri and Buchanan 2003).

Children with involved fathers fare better in school. A survey by the National Center for Education Statistics (1997) found that children with involved fathers are more likely to get mostly As, enjoy school, and participate in extracurricular activities. They are also less likely to repeat a grade.

8. Get Help

Many symptoms of depression and anxiety can be managed if you follow the steps listed above. However, if your symptoms don't resolve quickly or if they are severe, seek help from a trusted health care provider such as your family physician, or a qualified mental health professional such as a psychologist or psychiatrist. Often, consulting with a caring and knowledgeable professional can be the key to overcoming painful mood and anxiety symptoms.

Helping Her: How to Support Your Partner

Emotional difficulties in women during pregnancy and after delivery are surprisingly common. For example, studies consistently show that approximately 14 percent of women suffer from postpartum depression (Paulson, Dauber, and Leiferman 2006). In addition, some studies have found around 16 percent of women will experience clinically significant anxiety symptoms after delivery (Wenzel et al. 2005). Therefore, there's a good possibility that your partner will struggle with one or more of these emotional issues while pregnant or following the birth of your child.

If your partner is struggling with anxiety or depression, you may feel lost and confused. You want to know how you can help. Below, we've listed five key ways you can provide some much-needed support to your partner as the two of you become parents.

Empathize

Pregnancy and new motherhood is a time of tremendous change for women. During this time, she's experiencing physical and emotional changes, she's terrified about her new responsibilities, and she's fearful that her performance as a mother will be inadequate. It is difficult to see your partner going through this experience, and you may feel helpless to make things better. You may try to help her feel better, but your attempts to "fix" things will often be rejected (Morgan et al. 1997). Rather than becoming frustrated that your efforts to solve problems are not always appreciated, know that one of the best strategies you can use at this time is to just listen and hear how difficult things are for her. Simply let her know you care for her, and that you will go through this with her.

Know What to Watch Out For

Your partner may have the symptoms of anxiety listed in chapter 3 and throughout this book, such as panic attacks, obsessive thoughts, compulsive behaviors, or excessive worry. Or she may have the symptoms of postpartum depression listed earlier in this chapter. As a result, she may lose interest in interacting with her child or may tend only to the baby while completely neglecting her own needs. Although it's important not to overreact to minor symptoms, such as occasional crying or sadness, if your partner exhibits symptoms of anxiety or depression most of the day for a week or two, take action, because it may be a sign of a more serious problem.

If your partner is suffering from depression or anxiety, you might wonder why she's feeling that way. After all, having a child may be something she desperately wanted. The two of you may have gone to great lengths to get pregnant. And there's certainly a lot of joy that comes with a child. These factors may make your partner's negative emotions all the more puzzling and frustrating.

Although no one knows for sure why some new moms get depressed or anxious, researchers have uncovered some risk factors (Robertson et al. 2004), including the following:

- Depression during pregnancy

- Anxiety during pregnancy

- Stressful life events during pregnancy or shortly after delivery

- Lack of social support

- History of anxiety or depression

Pay particular attention if your partner has one or more of these risk factors. You can also discuss these risk factors with her. Of course, your partner can also develop anxiety or depression without these risk factors, so be on the lookout for symptoms. Encourage her to talk with her physician if you're concerned.

Get Help

If you have a partner who is suffering from postpartum anxiety or depression, help her get appropriate treatment from a medical or mental health professional. It may be tempting to go it alone and try to solve her problems on your own, but remember that postpartum anxiety and depression are real—and treatable—medical conditions and should be addressed as such. Just as you wouldn't try to treat any other serious illness yourself, you should not try to deal with your partner's postpartum anxiety and depression symptoms without the guidance of a health care provider.

What about suicide? The grim truth is that new moms suffering from postpartum depression are at significant risk for committing suicide. If you suspect that your partner may be having thoughts of suicide, get help immediately. If the danger is imminent, call 911 or get her to the nearest emergency room.

Help Out

As renowned relationship expert John Gottman (1999) wrote in his best-selling book *The Seven Principles for Making Marriage Work,* "Men have to do more housework!" Household help is particularly needed during the pregnancy and postpartum period. These are especially busy times: cribs need assembling, diapers need changing, clothes need folding, and bottles need washing. Believe it or not, simply doing more around the house can go a long way toward providing much-needed support for your partner.

Helping out can take many forms. Here are some specific ways you can give Mom a hand:

- Change diapers

- Feed your baby

- Prepare a meal

- Do the dishes

- Take the garbage out

- Shop for groceries

- Return phone calls

- Do laundry

- Clean the bathroom

Bond with Your Baby

How do some moms build that unbreakable bond with their children? The answer is simple. They form that connection by responding, moment by moment, to their child's needs. In other words, they focus intensely on caring and responding to their child.

Connecting with your child in this way is known as *attachment parenting* (Sears and Sears 2001) and it's one of the best things you can do for your child, yourself, and your spouse. And the good news is that attachment parenting isn't just for moms. Dads too can take advantage of this method of caring for your child. The only rule is to respond quickly and effectively to your child's need for food, comfort, stimulation, and physical contact. So hold your baby. Talk to her. Sing to her. Pick her up when she cries. Feed her when she's hungry. Rock her to sleep. Read a story to her. Give her a massage. Play with her. Bathe her. By giving her this intense attention, you'll be building a bond with your child, moment by moment, that will last a lifetime. You'll also be helping your partner by encouraging your child to attach to you as well as Mom.

A Coping Guide for Fathers

Helping Yourself

1. **Use This Book.** You can use the techniques listed in part 2 of this book to manage your own symptoms of anxiety.

2. **Consider the Benefits.** Keep in mind the reasons you decided to have a child. Write them down and review them often.

3. **Generate Coping Thoughts.** Make a list of thoughts that can help you cope when the going gets tough. For example, you might remind yourself that "This is only a phase," or "The baby is not doing it on purpose."

4. **Get Support.** Social support is crucial to coping with a new child. Identify your key sources of support and schedule time with them on a regular basis.

5. **Get Some Sleep.** Feeling well rested goes a long way toward minimizing feelings of depression and anxiety.

6. **Boost Your Skills.** Learn to be a better dad and you'll experience less depression and anxiety and feel more confident and competent.

7. **Know That Dads Matter.** Involved dads give their kids significant cognitive, emotional, and academic advantages.

8. **Get Help.** If you find that your symptoms don't resolve, seek help from a qualified professional.

Supporting Your Partner

1. **Empathize.** Focus on emotional support. Your attempts to "fix" things will often be rejected; your partner may be looking for empathy rather than a "solution" to her problem.

2. **Know What to Look For.** Symptoms of depression include depressed mood, lack of interest in previously enjoyable activities, frequent crying, weight loss, insomnia, and excessive guilt. Your partner might also experience panic attacks, obsessions, compulsions, and worry.

3. **Get Help.** If your partner is suffering from anxiety or depression, resist the urge to try to solve the problem on your own. Seek help from a qualified professional, such as a physician or a psychologist instead. If you suspect your partner is suicidal, seek help immediately.

4. **Help Out.** Take some heat off of Mom by lending a hand around the house. Fold laundry, do the dishes, take the garbage out, and so on.

5. **Bond with Your Baby.** Intense focus on your child's needs, through activities such as feeding, playing, and talking, encourages her to attach to you and will help build a bond that lasts a lifetime.

Key Points

- The pregnancy and postpartum period is stressful for fathers as well. This stress can make you particularly vulnerable to symptoms of depression or anxiety.

- If you do experience significant depression or anxiety symptoms, use the steps in this chapter to manage your symptoms, or seek help from a qualified mental health professional.

- If your partner is suffering from postpartum depression or anxiety, you can play a key role in her recovery.

- Although you can't cure your partner if she's suffering from postpartum depression or anxiety, you can help by understanding what she's experiencing, looking out for signs of more severe problems, seeking professional help if needed, helping out around the house, and bonding with your child.

Beyond Anxiety:
Postpartum Depression

We wrote this book to provide you with state-of-the-art strategies for overcoming anxiety during pregnancy and the postpartum period. However, this book wouldn't be complete without a word on postpartum depression. Depression and anxiety are kind of like thunder and lightning—they just go together. So, if you picked up this book because you're suffering from anxiety, then there's a good chance that you're experiencing at least some symptoms of depression as well.

Are You Depressed?

Since anxiety and depression often appear together, it can help for you to familiarize yourself with the symptoms of depression as you work on conquering your anxiety problem. Take a look at the list below and check off any symptoms (American Psychiatric Association 2000) that you've experienced recently:

☐ Persistently depressed mood

☐ Lack of interest in activities

☐ Significant weight loss or weight gain

☐ Difficulty sleeping or sleeping too much

☐ Fatigue or loss of energy

☐ Strong feelings of guilt or worthlessness

☐ Difficulty concentrating or trouble making decisions

☐ Spontaneous crying

☐ Lack of interest in your baby

☐ Thoughts of death or suicide

Note: *Postpartum depression significantly increases your risk of committing suicide. If you are having thoughts of taking your own life, please get help immediately.*

Mothers of newborns can expect some emotional symptoms during the postpartum period. Many women experience symptoms such as spontaneous crying during the first few days following delivery. This expected emotional reaction is commonly known as the "baby blues." These symptoms usually resolve within three to seven days after delivery (American Psychiatric Association 2000). However, for an estimated 14 percent of women, these symptoms will continue or worsen, leading to postpartum depression (Paulson, Dauber, and Leiferman 1996). If you've had any of the above symptoms and they've lasted longer than a few days, you may be suffering from postpartum depression.

What You Should Do Now

If you're experiencing symptoms of depression you might wonder what to do. First, be sure to discuss your symptoms of depression with your obstetrician or physician. That way the two of you can work together to create the safest and most effective treatment plan for you and your child. Also, if you're currently in cognitive behavioral therapy, discuss your depression symptoms with your therapist so the two of you can tailor your therapy to address depression as well as anxiety. If you are not in therapy, consider referring to the resource list near the end of this book to help you find an appropriate treatment provider or self-help materials that can help you get started overcoming your symptoms of depression.

Resources

In this section, we've included lists of additional resources that you may find helpful as you work on controlling your anxiety. You'll find self-help resources, websites, hotlines, and guides to finding professional help.

Self-Help Materials

Below we've listed some self-help resources. You may find the information and techniques described by these sources as a useful adjunct to this book.

Books

Anxiety and Depression

When Words Are Not Enough: The Women's Prescription for Depression and Anxiety by Valerie Davis Raskin

Beyond the Blues: A Guide to Understanding and Treating Prenatal and Postpartum Depression by Shoshana S. Bennett and Pec Indman

Mind Over Mood by Dennis Greenberger and Christine Padesky

This Isn't What I Expected: Overcoming Postpartum Depression by Karen Kleiman and Valerie Raskin

10 Simple Solutions to Worry: How to Calm Your Mind, Relax Your Body and Reclaim Your Life by Kevin L. Gyoerkoe and Pamela S. Wiegartz

The Anxiety and Phobia Workbook, fourth edition, by Edmund J. Bourne

General Pregnancy or Childcare

Mayo Clinic Guide to a Healthy Pregnancy by Mayo Clinic

Caring for Your Baby and Young Child: Birth to Age Five by the American Academy of Pediatrics

The Baby Book by William Sears, Martha Sears, Robert Sears, and James Sears

Websites

Postpartum Support International, www.postpartum.net

Anxiety Disorders Association of America, (ADAA), www.adaa.org

Postpartum Progress, www.postpartumprogress.typepad.com

March of Dimes, www.marchofdimes.com

Hotlines

Postpartum Support International, 800-944-4PPD (800-944-4773)

National Suicide Prevention Lifeline, 800-273-TALK (800-273-8255)

How to Find Professional Help

In the section below, we've listed ways to find trained, professional help for your symptoms of anxiety or depression. If you think you'd benefit from professional help, you can use the resources listed below to help you find a professional that best fits your needs.

Cognitive Behavioral Therapy

Anxiety Disorders Association of America (ADAA), www.adaa.org

Association for Behavioral and Cognitive Therapies (ABCT), www.abct.org

Medication Management

MedEdPPD Provider Search Directory, www.mededppd.org/mothers/referral_center.asp

Postpartum Progress, postpartumprogress.typepad.com/weblog/postpartum-depression-anxiety-psychosis-treatment-program.html

The Motherisk ReproPsych Group, www.motherisk.org/prof/reproPsych.jsp

Pre- or Postnatal Care

American College of Obstetricians and Gynecologists, www.acog.org

National Women's Health Information Center, 800-994-9662, www.womenshealth.gov

References

Abramowitz, J., K. Moore, C. Carmin, P. S. Wiegartz, and C. Purdon. 2001. Acute onset of obsessive compulsive disorder in males following childbirth. *Psychosomatics* 42:429–31.

Abramowitz, J. S., S. Schwartz, and K. M. Moore. 2003. Obsessional thoughts in postpartum females and their partners: Content, severity and relationship with depression. *Journal of Clinical Psychology in Medical Settings* 10 (3):157–64.

Abramowitz, J. S., S. A. Schwartz, K. M. Moore, and K. R. Luenzmann. 2003. Obsessive-compulsive symptoms in pregnancy and the puerperium: A review of the literature. *Anxiety Disorders,* 17:461–78.

Adewuya, A. O., B. A. Ola, O. O. Aloba, and B. M. Mapayi. 2006. Anxiety disorders among Nigerian women in late pregnancy: A controlled study. *Archives of Women's Mental Health* 9 (6): 325–28.

Altemus, M., J. Fong, R. Yang, S. Damast, V. Luine, and D. Ferguson. 2004. Changes in cerebrospinal fluid neurochemistry during pregnancy. *Biological Psychiatry* 56:386–92.

Altemus, M., and K. Brogan. 2004. Pregnancy and postpartum. *Scientific Symposium Monograph* Suppl:10–11.

American Psychiatric Association. 2000. *Diagnostic and Statistical Manual of Mental Disorders* (DSM-IV-TR). 4th ed. Text rev. Washington, DC: American Psychiatric Association.

Armstrong, K. L., A. R. Van Haeringen, M. R. Dadds, and R. Cash. 1998. Sleep deprivation or postnatal depression in later infancy: Separating the chicken from the egg. *Journal of Pediatrics and Child Health* 34 (3): 260–62.

Austin, M-P., M. Frilingos, J. Lumley, D. Hadzi-Pavlovic, W. Roncolato, S. Acland, K. Saint, N. Segal, and G. Parker. 2008. Brief antenatal cognitive behaviour therapy group intervention for the prevention of postnatal depression and anxiety: A randomised controlled trial. *Journal of Affective Disorders* 105:35–44.

Austin, M-P., D. Hadzi-Pavlovic, L. Leader, K. Saint, and G. Parker. 2005. Maternal trait anxiety, depression and life event stress in pregnancy: Relationships with infant temperament. *Early Human Development* 81 (2): 183–90.

Austin, M-P., L. Tully, and G. Parker. 2007. Examining the relationship between antenatal anxiety and postnatal depression. *Journal of Affective Disorders* 101:169–74.

Ayers, S., and A. D. Pickering. 2001. Do women get posttraumatic stress disorder as a result of childbirth? A prospective study of incidence. *Birth* 28 (2): 111–18.

Baer, L. 2001. *The Imp of the Mind: Exploring the Silent Epidemic of Obsessive Bad Thoughts.* New York: Plume.

Balaji, A. B., A. H. Claussen, D. C. Smith, S. N. Visser, M. J. Morales, and R. Perou. 2007. Social support networks and maternal mental health and well-being. *Journal of Women's Health* 16 (10): 1386–96.

Beck, J. 1995. *Cognitive Therapy: Basics and Beyond.* New York: Guilford Press.

Berle, J. O., A. Mykletun, A. K. Daltveit, S. Rasmussen, F. Holsten, and A. A. Dahl. 2005. Neonatal outcomes in offspring of women with anxiety and depression during pregnancy. *Archives of Women's Mental Health* 8 (3): 181–89.

Breitkopf, C. R., L. A. Primeau, R. E. Levine, G. L. Olson, Z. H. Wu, and A. B. Berenson. 2006. Anxiety symptoms during pregnancy and postpartum. *Journal of Psychosomatic Obstetrics and Gynecology.* 27 (3): 157–62.

Brisch, K. H., D. Munz, H. Kachele, R. Terinde, and R. Kreienberg. 2005. Effects of previous pregnancy loss on level of maternal anxiety after prenatal ultrasound screening for fetal malformation. *Journal of Loss and Trauma* 10 (2): 131–53.

Brockington, I. F., E. Macdonald, and G. Wainscott. 2006. Anxiety, obsessions, and morbid preoccupations in pregnancy and the puerperium. *Archives of Women's Mental Health* 9 (5): 253–63.

Brown, T. A., T. A. O'Leary, and D. H. Barlow. 2001. Generalized anxiety disorder. In *Clinical Handbook of Psychological Disorders,* 3rd ed., edited by D. H. Barlow. New York: Guilford Press.

Burns, D. D. 1999. *Feeling Good: The New Mood Therapy.* Rev. ed. New York: HarperCollins.

———. 2006. *When Panic Attacks: The New, Drug-Free Anxiety Therapy That Can Change Your Life.* New York: Morgan Road Books.

Carter, C. S., M. Altemus, and G. P. Chrousos. 2001. Neuroendocrine and emotional changes in the postpartum period. *Progress in Brain Research* 133:241–49.

Chambless, D. L., and M. M. Gillis. 1993. Cognitive therapy of anxiety disorders. *Journal of Consulting and Clinical Psychology* 61 (2): 248–60.

Coates, A. O., C. A. Schaefer, and J. L. Alexander. 2004. Detection of postpartum depression and anxiety in a large health plan. *Journal of Behavioral Health Services and Research* 31 (2): 117–33.

Cobb, S. 1976. Social support as a moderator of life stress. *Psychosomatic Medicine* 38: 300–314.

Cohen, L. S., D. A. Sichel, J. A. Dimmock, and J. F. Rosenbaum. 1994. Postpartum course in women with preexisting panic disorder. *Journal of Clinical Psychiatry* 55 (7): 289–92.

Coleman, V., M. Carter, M. Morgan, and J. Schulkin. 2008. Obstetrician-gynecologists' screening patterns for anxiety during pregnancy. *Depression and Anxiety* 25 (2): 114–23.

Coplan, R. J., K. O'Neil, and K. A. Arbeau. 2005. Maternal anxiety during and after pregnancy and infant temperament at three months of age. *Journal of Prenatal and Perinatal Psychology and Health* 19 (3): 199–215.

Cosby, B. *Fatherhood.* 1987. New York: Berkley Trade.

Craske, M. G., R. M. Rapee, L. Jackel, and D. H. Barlow. 1989. Qualitative dimensions of worry in DSM-III-R generalized anxiety disorder subjects and nonanxious controls. *Behavior Research and Therapy* 27:397–402.

Creedy, D. K., I. M. Schochet, and J. Horsfall. 2000. Childbirth and the development of acute trauma symptoms: Incidence and contributing factors. *Birth: Issues in Perinatal Care* 27 (2): 104–111.

David, E. P., N. Snidman, P. D. Wadhwa, L. M. Glynn, C. D. Schetter, and C. A. Sandman. 2004. Prenatal maternal anxiety and depression predict negative behavioral reactivity in infancy. *Infancy* 6 (3): 319–31.

Dayan, J., C. Creveuil, M. N. Marks, S. Conroy, M. Herlicoviez, M. Dreyfus, and S. Tordjman. 2006. Prenatal depression, prenatal anxiety, and spontaneous preterm birth: A prospective cohort study among women with early and regular care. *Psychosomatic Medicine* 68 (6): 938–46.

Dennis, C-L., and L. Ross. 2006. Women's perceptions of partner support and conflict in the development of postpartum depressive symptoms. *Journal of Advanced Nursing* 56: 588–99.

Dugas, M. J., and R. Ladouceur. 2000. Treatment of GAD: Targeting intolerance of uncertainty in two types of worry. *Behavior Modification* 24 (5): 635–57.

Elliott, T. R., R. Shewchuk, C. Richeson, H. Pickelman, and K. W. Franklin. 1996. Problem-solving and the prediction of depression during pregnancy and in the postpartum period. *Journal of Counseling and Development* 74: 645–51.

Fairbrother, N., and S. R. Woody. 2008. New mothers' thoughts of harm related to the newborn. *Archives of Women's Mental Health* 11: 221–29.

Faisal-Cury, A., and P. R. Menezes. 2007. Prevalence of anxiety and depression during pregnancy in a private setting sample. *Archives of Women's Mental Health* 10 (1): 25–32.

Flouri, E., and A. Buchanan. 2003. The role of father involvement in children's later mental health. *Journal of Adolescence* 26 (1): 63–78.

Foa, E. B., and M. J. Kozak. 1986. Emotional processing of fear: Exposure to corrective information. *Psychological Bulletin* 99: 20–35.

Foa, E. B., B. O. Rothbaum, D. S. Riggs, and T. B. Murdock. 1991. Treatment of posttraumatic stress disorder in rape victims: A comparison between cognitive-behavioral procedures and counseling. *Journal of Consulting and Clinical Psychology* 59: 715–23.

Franklin, M. E., Riggs, D. S., and Pai, A. 2005. Obsessive-compulsive disorder. In *Improving Outcomes and Preventing Relapses in Cognitive-Behavioral Therapy*, edited by M. M. Antony, D. R. Ledley, and R. G. Heimberg. New York: Guilford Press.

Geller, P. A., D. Kerns, and C. M. Klier. 2004. Anxiety following miscarriage and the subsequent pregnancy: A review of the literature and future directions. *Journal of Psychosomatic Research* 56 (1): 35–45.

Glazier, R. H., F. J. Elgar, V. Goel, and S. Holzapfel. 2004. Stress, social support and emotional distress in a community sample of pregnant women. *Journal of Psychosomatic Obstetrics and Gynecology* 25: 247–55.

Gottman, J. 1999. *The Seven Principles for Making Marriage Work.* New York: Three Rivers Press.

Grant, K-A., C. McMahon, and M-P. Austin. 2008. Maternal anxiety during the transition to parenthood: A prospective study. *Journal of Affective Disorders* 108: 101–111.

Gyoerkoe, K. L., and P. S. Wiegartz. 2006. *10 Simple Solutions to Worry: How to Calm Your Mind, Relax Your Body, and Reclaim Your Life.* Oakland, CA: New Harbinger Publications.

Heron, J., T. G. O'Connor, J. Evans, J. Golding, and V. Glover. 2004. The course of anxiety and depression through pregnancy and the postpartum in a community sample. *Journal of Affective Disorders* 80 (1): 65–73.

Hertzberg, T., and K. Wahlbeck. 1999. The impact of pregnancy and puerperium on panic disorder: a review. *Journal of Psychosomatic Obstetrics and Gynecology* 20: 59–64.

House, J. S. 1981. *Work Stress and Social Support.* Reading, MA: Addison-Wesley.

Jacobson, E. 1929. *Progressive Relaxation.* Chicago: University of Chicago Press.

Kelly, M., and B. B. Little. 2001. Obstetrics for the non-obstetrician. In *Management of Psychiatric Disorders in Pregnancy,* edited by K. Yonkers and B. Little. London: Arnold.

Kelly, R. H., J. Russo, and W. Katon. 2001. Somatic complaints among pregnant women cared for in obstetrics: Normal pregnancy or depressive and anxiety symptom amplification revisited? *General Hospital Psychiatry* 23 (3): 107–113.

Kelly, R. H., D. F. Zatzick, and T. F. Anders. 2001. The detection and treatment of psychiatric disorders and substance use among pregnant women cared for in obstetrics. *American Journal of Psychiatry* 158 (2): 213–19.

Kendell, R. E., J. C. Chalmers, and C. L. Platz. 1987. Epidemiology of puerperal psychoses. *British Journal of Psychiatry* 150: 662–73.

Keogh, E., S. Ayers, and H. Francis. 2002. Does anxiety sensitivity predict post-traumatic stress symptoms following childbirth? A preliminary report. *Cognitive Behaviour Therapy* 31 (4): 145–55.

Kessler, R. C., K. A. McGonagle, S. Zhao, C. B. Nelson, M. Hughes, S. Eshelman et al. 1994. Lifetime and twelve-month prevalence of DSM-III-R psychiatric disorders in the United States: Results from the national comorbidity survey. *Archives of General Psychiatry* 51:8–19.

Kessler, R. C., A. Sonnega, E. Bromet, and C. B. Nelson. 1995. Posttraumatic stress disorder in the National Comorbidity Study. *Archives of General Psychiatry* 52:1048–60.

Kleiner, S. M., and B. Condor. 2007. *The Good Mood Diet.* New York: Springboard Press.

Labad, J., J. M. Menchon, P. Alonso, C. Segalas, S. Jimenez, and J. Vallejo. 2005. Female reproductive cycle and obsessive-compulsive disorder. *Journal of Clinical Psychiatry* 66:428–35.

Ladouceur, R., P. Gosselin, and M. J. Dugas. 2000. Experimental manipulation of intolerance of uncertainty: A study of a theoretical model of worry. *Behaviour Research and Therapy* 38 (9): 933–41.

Leahy, R. 2003. *Cognitive Therapy Techniques: A Practitioner's Guide.* New York: Guilford Press.

Long, B. C., and van Stavel, R. 1995. Effects of exercise training on anxiety: A meta-analysis. *Journal of Applied Sport Psychology* 7 (2): 167–189.

Lovestone, S., and R. Kumar. 1993. Postnatal psychiatric illness: the impact on partners. *British Journal of Psychiatry* 163: 210–16.

Mancuso, R. A., C. D. Schetter, C. M. Rini, S. C. Roesch, and C. J. Hobel. 2004. Maternal prenatal anxiety and corticotrophin-releasing hormone associated with timing of delivery. *Psychosomatic Medicine* 66 (5): 762–69.

Matthey, S., B. Barnett, D. J. Kavanagh, and P. Howie. 2001. Validation of the Edinburgh Postnatal Depression Scale for men, and comparison of item endorsement with their partners. *Journal of Affective Disorders* 64:175–84.

Matthey, S., B. Barnett, P. Howie, and D. J. Kavanagh. 2003. Diagnosing postpartum depression in mothers and fathers: Whatever happened to anxiety? *Journal of Affective Disorders* 74 (2): 139–47.

Mayo Clinic. 2004. *Mayo Clinic Guide to a Healthy Pregnancy.* New York: Harper Collins.

McCabe, R. E., and M. M. Antony. 2005. Panic Disorder and Agoraphobia. In *Improving Outcomes and Preventing Relapses in Cognitive-Behavioral Therapy*, edited by M. M. Antony, D. R. Ledley, and R. G. Heimberg. New York: Guilford Press.

McKay, M, P. D. Rogers, and J. McKay. 2003. *When Anger Hurts: Quieting the Storm Within.* 2nd ed. Oakland, CA: New Harbinger Publications.

Mezzacappa, E. S., W. Guethlein, N. Vaz, and E. Begiella. 2000. A preliminary study of breast-feeding and maternal symptomatology. *Annals of Behavioral Medicine* 22:71–79.

Morgan, M., S. Matthey, B. Barnett, and C. Richardson. 1997. A group programme for postnatally distressed women and their partners. *Journal of Advanced Nursing* 26 (5): 913–20.

National Center for Education Statistics. 1997. Fathers' involvement in their children's schools. www .nces.ed.gov (accessed July 30, 2008).

Northcott, C. J., and M. B. Stein. 1994. Panic disorder in pregnancy. *Journal of Clinical Psychiatry* 55 (12): 539–42.

Nonacs, R. M., L. S. Cohen, A. C. Viguera, and J. Mogielnicki. 2005. Diagnosis and treatment of mood and anxiety disorders in pregnancy. In *Mood and Anxiety Disorders During Pregnancy and Postpartum,* edited by L. S. Cohen and R. M. Nonacs. Washington, DC: American Psychiatric Publishing.

Norton, G. R., J. Dorward, and B.J. Cox. 1986. Factors associated with panic attacks in nonclinical subjects. *Behavior Therapy* 17 (3): 239–52.

O'Connor, T. G., J. Heron, and V. Glover. 2002. Antenatal anxiety predicts child behavioral/emotional problems independently of postnatal depression. *Journal of the American Academy of Child and Adolescent Psychiatry* 41 (12): 1470–77.

Orr, S. T., J. P. Reiter, D. G. Blazer, and S. A. James. 2007. Maternal prenatal pregnancy-related anxiety and spontaneous preterm birth in Baltimore, Maryland. *Psychosomatic Medicine* 69 (6): 566–70.

Paulson, J. F., S. Dauber, and J. A. Leiferman. 2006. Individual and Combined Effects of Postpartum Depression in Mothers and Fathers on Parenting Behavior. *Pediatrics* 118:659–68.

Radin, N. 1994. Primary-caregiving fathers in intact families. In *Redefining Families: Implications for Children's Development,* edited by A. E. Gottfried and A. W. Gottfried. New York: Plume.

Raikes, H. A., and R. A. Thompson. 2005. Efficacy and social support as predictors of parenting stress among families in poverty. *Infant Mental Health Journal* 26:177–90.

Robertson, E., S. Grace, T. Wallington, and D. E. Stewart. 2004. Antenatal risk factors for postpartum depression: A synthesis of recent literature. *General Hospital Psychiatry* 26 (4): 289–95.

Rogal, S. S., K. Poschman, K. Belanger, H. B. Howell, M. V. Smith, J. Medina, and K. A. Yonkers. 2007. Effects of posttraumatic stress disorder on pregnancy outcomes. *Journal of Affective Disorders* 102:137–143.

Ross, L. E., and L. M. McLean. 2006. Anxiety disorders during pregnancy and the postpartum period: A systematic review. *Journal of Clinical Psychiatry* 67 (8): 1285–98.

Salkovskis, P. M. 1999. Understanding and treating obsessive-compulsive disorder. *Behaviour Research and Therapy* 37:S29–S52.

Sampson, S. 2001. Being female and anxious: Anxiety disorders in women. *ADAA Reporter* 12 (3): 1, 8–9.

Sayil, M., A. Gure, and Z. Ucanok. 2007. First time mothers' anxiety and depressive symptoms across the transition to motherhood: Associations with maternal and environmental characteristics. *Women and Health* 44:61–77.

Sears, W., and M. Sears. 2001. *The Attachment Parenting Book: A Commonsense Guide to Understanding and Nurturing Your Baby.* New York: Little, Brown.

Shields, B. 2005. *Down Came the Rain.* New York: Hyperion.

Sholomskas, D. E., P. J. Wickamaratne, L. Dogolo, D.W. O'Brien, P. J. Leaf, and S. W. Woods. 1993. Postpartum onset of panic disorder: a coincidental event? *Journal of Clinical Psychiatry* 54:476–80.

Smith, M. V., K. Poschman, M. A. Caveleri, H. B. Howell, and K. A.Yonkers. 2006. Symptoms of posttraumatic stress disorder in a community sample of low-income pregnant women. *American Journal of Psychiatry* 163 (5): 881–84.

Smith, M. V., R. A. Rosenheck, M. A.Cavaleri, H. B. Howell, K. Poschman, and K. Yonkers. 2004. Screening for and detection of Depression, Panic Disorder, and PTSD in public-sector obstetric clinics. *Psychiatric Services* 55 (4): 407–414.

Sutter-Dallay, A. L., V. Giaconne-Marcesche, E. Glatigny-Dally, and H. Verdoux. 2004. Women with anxiety disorders during pregnancy are at increased risk of intense postnatal depressive symptoms: A prospective survey of the MATQUID cohort. *European Psychiatry* 19 (8): 459–63.

Taylor, S., D. S. Thordarson, L. Maxfield, I. C. Federoff, K. Lovell, and J. Ogrodiczuk. 2003. Comparative efficacy, speed, and adverse effects of three PTSD treatments: Exposure therapy, EMDR, and relaxation training. *Journal of Consulting and Clinical Psychology* 71 (2): 330–38.

Teixeira, J., D. Martin, O. Prendiville, and V. Glover. 2005. The effects of acute relaxation on indices of anxiety during pregnancy. *Journal of Psychosomatic Obstetrics and Gynecology* 26 (4): 271–76.

Uguz, F. K., C. Akman, N. Kaya, and A. S. Cilli. 2007. Postpartum-onset obsessive-compulsive disorder: Incidence, clinical features, and related factors. *Journal of Clinical Psychiatry* 68: 132–38.

Uguz, F. K., K. Gezginc, I. E. Zeytinci, S. Karatayli, R. Askin, O. Guler, F. K. Sahin, H. M. Emul, O. Ozbulut, and O. Gecici. 2007. Obsessive-compulsive disorder in pregnant women during the third trimester of pregnancy. *Comprehensive Psychiatry* 48:441–45.

Van den Bergh, B. R. H., M. Mennes, J. Oosterlaan, V. Stevens, P. Stiers, A. Marcoen, and L. Lagae. 2005. High antenatal maternal anxiety is related to impulsivity during performance on cognitive tasks in fourteen- and fifteen-year-olds. *Neuroscience and Biobehavioral Reviews.* 29 (2): 259–69.

Van Eerde, W. 2003. Procrastination at work and time management training. *Journal of Psychology* 137 (5): 421–34.

Vliegen, N., P. Luyten, P. Meurs, and G. Cluckers. 2006. Adaptive and maladaptive dimensions of relatedness and self-definition: Relationship with postpartum depression and anxiety. *Personality and Individual Differences* 41 (3): 395–406.

Vulink, N. C. C., D. Denys, L. Bus, and H. G. M. Westenberg. 2006. Female hormones affect symptom severity in obsessive-compulsive disorder. *International Clinical Psychopharmacology* 21:171–75.

Wegman, D. 1994. *White Bears and Other Unwanted Thoughts: Suppression, Obsession, and the Psychology of Mental Control.* New York: Guilford Press.

Wenzel, A., E. N. Haugen, L. C. Jackson, and J. R. Brendle. 2005. Anxiety symptoms and disorders at eight weeks postpartum. *Anxiety Disorders* 19:295–311.

Zachariah, R. 2004. Attachment, social support, life stress and psychological well-being in pregnant low-income women: A pilot study. *Clinical Excellence for Nurse Practitioners* 8 (2): 60–62.

Pamela S. Wiegartz, Ph.D., was an associate professor at the University of Illinois at Chicago where she taught courses on cognitive behavioral therapy (CBT) and directed the obsessive-compulsive disorder (OCD) clinic for over a decade. She is a certified fellow of the Academy of Cognitive Therapy and serves on the scientific advisory board of OCD Chicago. Wiegartz is also actively involved in clinical research and is a cognitive behavioral consultant on grant-funded projects related to perinatal depression management and self-care. A licensed clinical psychologist, she maintains a practice dedicated to treating individuals with anxiety disorders in the greater Boston area. She is coauthor of *10 Simple Solutions to Worry*. Visit her online at www.anxietyandocdtreatment.com.

Kevin L. Gyoerkoe, Psy.D., is codirector of the Anxiety and Agoraphobia Treatment Center, a clinic specializing in treating anxiety with cognitive behavioral therapy (CBT). He is an assistant professor at the Chicago School of Professional Psychology, where he teaches courses on CBT. Gyoerkoe is certified by the Academy of Cognitive Therapy and serves on the scientific advisory board of OCD Chicago. He is coauthor of *10 Simple Solutions to Worry*.

Foreword writer **Laura J. Miller, MD**, is a professor of psychiatry at the University of Illinois, Chicago (UIC), and associate head of its department of psychiatry. She is director of the UIC Women's Mental Health Program and winner of the American Psychiatric Association's Gold Achievement Award for innovative mental health services and the American College of Psychiatrists' Award for creativity in psychiatric education. Miller is also director of the Illinois Peripartum Mental Health Project. She has published over sixty articles and book chapters related to women's mental health and edited the book *Postpartum Mood Disorders*.

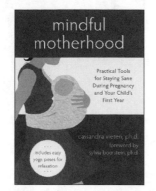
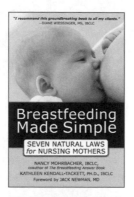
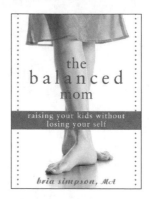
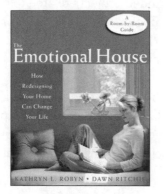
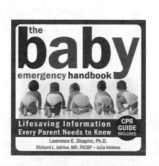
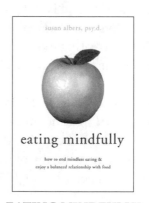